EMS

and the Law

EMS

and the Law

American Academy of Orthopaedic Surgeons
Authors:
Jacob L. Hafter, NREMT-P, MS, Esq.
Victoria L. Fedor, NREMT-P, Esq.

JONES AND BARTLETT PUBLISHERS
Sudbury, Massachusetts
BOSTON   TORONTO   LONDON   SINGAPORE

THE RICHARD STOCKTON COLLEGE
OF NEW JERSEY LIBRARY
POMONA, NEW JERSEY 08240-0195

Jones and Bartlett Publishers

World Headquarters
40 Tall Pine Drive
Sudbury, MA 01776
978-443-5000
info@jbpub.com
www.jbpub.com

Jones and Bartlett Publishers Canada
2406 Nikanna Road
Mississauga, ON L5C 2W6
CANADA

Jones and Bartlett Publishers International
Barb House, Barb Mews
London W6 7PA
United Kingdom

Production Credits

Chief Executive Officer: Clayton E. Jones
Chief Operating Officer: Donald W. Jones, Jr.
Executive V.P. and Publisher: Robert Holland
V.P. of Sales and Marketing: William J. Kane
V.P. Production and Design: Anne Spencer
V.P. Manufacturing and Inventory Control: Therese Bräuer
Publisher, Public Safety: Kimberly Brophy
Associate Editor: Elizabeth Petersen
Production Editor: Scarlett Stoppa
Director of Marketing: Alisha Weisman
Cover Design: Kristin Ohlin
Cover Photography: © PhotoDisc/Getty Images
Chapter Opener Images: © AbleStock
Typesetting: Carlisle Communications
Printing and Binding: DB Hess
Cover Printer: Lehigh Press

RICHARD STOCKTON COLLEGE

3 3005 00706 9917

American Academy of Orthopaedic Surgeons

Editorial Credits

Chief Education Officer: Mark W. Wieting
Director, Department of Publications: Marilyn L. Fox, PhD
Managing Editor: Lynne Roby Shindoll
Senior Editor: Barbara A. Scotese

Board of Directors 2003

James H. Herndon, MD, President
Robert W. Bucholz, MD
Stuart Weinstein, MD
Vernon T. Tolo, MD
Richard H. Gelberman, MD
E. Anthony Rankin, MD
Edward A. Toriello, MD
Stephen A. Albanese, MD
Frederick M. Azar, MD
Laura L. Tosi, MD
Gerald R. Williams, Jr., MD
Maureen Finnegan, MD
Peter J. Mandell, MD
David G. Lewallen, MD
Glenn B. Pfeffer, MD
Mark C. Gebhardt, MD
Leslie L. Altick
Karen L. Hackett, FACHE, CAE (*Ex Officio*)

Copyright © 2004 Jones and Bartlett Publishers, Inc.

All rights reserved. No part of the material protected by this copyright may be reproduced or utilized in any form, electronic or mechanical, including photocopying, recording, or by any information storage and retrieval system, without written permission from the copyright owner.

The procedures and protocols in this book are based on the most current recommendations of responsible medical sources. The American Academy of Orthopaedic Surgeons and the publisher, however, make no guarantee as to, and assume no responsibility for, the correctness, sufficiency, or completeness of such information or recommendations. Other or additional safety measures may be required under particular circumstances.

This textbook is intended solely as a guide to the appropriate procedures to be employed when rendering emergency care to the sick and injured. It is not intended as a statement of the standards of care required in any particular situation, because circumstances and the patient's physical condition can vary widely from one emergency to another. Nor is it intended that this textbook shall in any way advise emergency personnel concerning legal authority to perform the activities or procedures discussed. Such local determinations should be made only with the aid of legal counsel.

Library of Congress Cataloging-in-Publication Data

Hafter, Jacob.
    EMS and the law / Jacob Hafter.-- 1st ed.
        p. ; cm.
Includes index.
    ISBN 0-7637-2068-2 (alk. paper)
1. Emergency medical services--Law and legislation--United States.
[DNLM: 1. Emergency Medical Services--legislation &
jurisprudence--United States. 2. Insurance, Liability--legislation &
jurisprudence--United States. 3. Malpractice--legislation &
jurisprudence--United States. 4. Patient Rights--legislation &
jurisprudence--United States. WX 33 AA1 H139e 2004] I. Title.
    KF3826.E5H34 2004
    344.7303'218--dc22

                                        2003023835

Printed in the United States of America
07 06 05 04 03   10 9 8 7 6 5 4 3 2 1

KF 3826 .E5 H34 2004
53369222
EMS and the law

Contents

THE RICHARD STOCKTON COLLEGE
OF NEW JERSEY LIBRARY
POMONA, NEW JERSEY 08240-0195

THE RICHARD STOCKTON COLLEGE
OF NEW JERSEY LIBRARY
P.O. NOVA, NEW JERSEY 08240-0195

Acknowledgments

Michael R. Kass, JD, MS, EMT-Basic was a contributing author for this text.

Jones and Bartlett Publishers would like to thank the following people for reviewing this text:

Spencer A. Hall, MD, JD, FCLM
Diplomate, American Board of Legal Medicine
Physician and Attorney at Law
Lincoln, New Mexico

Scot Phelps, JD, MPH, REMT-P
Sleepy Hollow, New York

Edward Pike, JD, EMT-P, I/C
Boston EMS
Boston, Massachusetts

Walk-Through

EMS and the Law

is a primer about the American legal system as it applies to EMS providers, offering a basic overview of laws and rights with detailed descriptions of how they affect EMS. No matter how well-trained or experienced an EMS provider is, legal issues are an ever-present concern.

This book will furnish EMS providers with a thorough understanding of lawsuits, patient and provider rights, HIPPA and other health care regulations, negligence, documentation, and more.

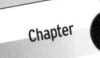

Special Features
- **You Be the Judge**—Brief case studies intended to demonstrate various legal principles and topics.
- **Legally Speaking**—Boxed features that provide quick definitions of essential legal terms.
- **Legal Practices**—Boxed features that provide legal tips for EMS providers.

Mechanics of the Legal System

You Be the Judge

An emergency medical technician (EMT) is responding to a call that requires him to drive through a school zone to reach the scene of the ill patient. It is 7:53 am, and the school crosswalk is filled with primary grade students walking towards the building. The posted speed limit is 20 mph. The EMT is driving at a rate of 29 mph, as recorded by the radar of the police officer monitoring the school zone. In accordance with system protocols and state law, the ambulance is traveling with full lights and sirens turned on. As the ambulance progresses through the crosswalk, it strikes and kills a 6-year-old student. The jury deliberating the case is composed of parents and grandparents.

How might the verdict of this case and its associated damages be determined?

The American legal system affects the emergency medical service (EMS) provider because it impacts his or her ability to deliver health care in an emergency situation. In the ever-changing world of EMS, it is difficult enough to keep up with the rapidly developing technological and medical advances without stopping to worry about the possibility of having to defend yourself in a lawsuit. This chapter explains the legal system and its historical application to EMS and examines future trends in EMS litigation.

Components of the American Legal System

The American legal system is defined, administered, and enforced by the government. The federal and state governments are divided into three distinct branches: the legislative branch, the executive branch, and the judicial branch. These branches of government have a daily impact on how EMS providers deliver care to the public.

In order for a bill to become a law, the legislative branch, as well as the chief executive of the executive branch, must approve it. The **legislative branch** consists of the legislature, the body of elected officials that creates and enacts laws. The federal legislature is made up of two separate

Legally Speaking

legislative branch The branch of the government containing the legislature; the elected officials who write and enact laws.

executive branch The branch of the government that reports directly to the chief executive; responsible for executing, administering, and seeking court or administrative enforcement of laws and regulations; federal agencies overseen by the executive branch, including the FDA, DEA, and OSHA; state agencies include Departments of Public Health and EMS licensing and regulatory boards.

judicial branch The branch of government containing the courts that enforce the law and resolve disputes based on analysis of what the law means and how it applies to a given situation.

state action An action or responsibility of the state government.

federal action An action or responsibility of the federal government.

entities: the Senate and the House of Representatives. The legislative branch of the federal government is known as Congress. Most, if not all, state legislatures are also made up of a state Senate and a state House of Representatives.

The legislature writes laws that govern EMS, including laws concerning certification and accreditation, medical control (the ongoing oversight of the physician under whose license the EMS facility operates), the staffing of ambulances, and the rules and regulations pertaining to emergency response vehicles. The legislature often defers specific EMS policy and rule making to an EMS administrative agency or advisory board. Such administrative agencies and boards report to, and are typically appointed by, the chief executive, such as a state's governor or the president of the United States. In addition to responding to legislative delegation, these administrative agencies create and enforce policies, including the regulation and oversight of the local and regional rule-making committees, advisory boards, and educational standards.

The **executive branch** of the government consists of all regulatory and enforcement agencies, boards, and commissions. This branch enforces the laws that are created by the legislative branch. The president of the United States is the chief executive of the federal government. The chief executive of each state's government is that state's governor. Examples of federal executive branch agencies that impact EMS include the Food and Drug Administration (FDA), the Occupational Safety and Health Administration (OSHA), and the Drug Enforcement Administration (DEA). State executive branch agencies include the medical licensing board, EMS regulatory agency or commission, and the Department of Public Health. The president and the governor appoint the directors of each of these agencies. They also appoint the members of regulatory boards and commissions that govern EMS. Therefore, in order for EMS providers to have a voice in the development of government policies, it is important for them to be politically active.

The **judicial branch** is the branch of government that contains all of the courts. The federal judicial branch is made up of all of the federal courts, including the highest court in the nation—the United States Supreme Court. The state's judicial branch is composed of all state courts. The mission of the federal and state level courts is to enforce the policies and procedures of the executive and legislative branches. Courts are also responsible for securing a safe and efficient forum to enforce laws and regulations and resolve disputes concerning the administration of such legislated laws and regulations.

EMS policies are primarily regulated by **state actions.** However, certain **federal actions** may also influence EMS. Some federal actions require state and local adherence; others are optional for states to follow. For example, the Department of Transportation (DOT), a federal agency, creates and publishes a national curriculum for EMTs. Each state can choose whether it will adopt the DOT curriculum as a state EMS standard. On the other hand, administrative rules and regulations put into effect by OSHA must be followed by all state and local EMS agencies. In general, if a state's requirements are higher or more stringent than the federal regulations, the state's requirements are followed.

The best way to understand the laws affecting EMS in a particular region is to look at that region's state statutes regulating EMS providers. The legislature within each state is responsible for developing laws that provide oversight for the EMS providers and their respective systems—the network of agreed upon policies and coordinated procedures between the basic life support and advanced life support ambulance providers, the first-responder fire and police departments, the hospitals, medical control, and communications and support services within a given locality. Whereas some states have created very thorough legislative provisions, others have enacted statutes that only cover the bare minimum of EMS regulation. **Table 1.1** provides a list of each state's legislative provisions. At the bottom of this table is a key to the symbols and abbreviations used. To obtain a copy of the text of the laws and regulations listed in this table, check the internet to see if your state has its laws online or contact your state's department of official publications. You should also be able to find copies of your state's laws at your local library.

Most states have purposely enacted vague or minimal statutory language. These vaguely written statutes are known as "enabling" statutes because they authorize, empower, or enable an administrative regulatory agency, board, or commission within the executive branch of the government to enact comprehensive rules and regulations for governing EMS practices that have the same force and effect of a general law. Such boards are usually made up of professionals from within the EMS field as well as representatives of EMS consumer groups and the general public. Members of the public are appointed to these boards to provide balance and ensure that the public's interests are protected.

States that have implemented such boards or agencies find this form of delegated rule-making to be efficient and effective because of the expertise of the members serving on the board. The advisory board usually has a higher level of knowledge and familiarity with EMS administration and state-specific EMS issues than the state legislators. The EMS advisory board can also spend more time than the state legislature addressing the issues that are most important to EMS. In addition, because the advisory board is composed of EMS professionals, the board-created rules and regulations have a better likelihood of being complied with than if they were created by elected politicians with varied backgrounds who may have received campaign contributions from hospitals or special interest groups that could potentially influence their stance on EMS-related issues.

Table 1.1

Listing of State EMS Statutes

Ala. Code § 22-18-1 to § 22-18-44 (Supp. 1999)
Alaska Stat. § 10.08.010 to § 18.08.090 (Supp. 1999)
Ariz. Rev. Stat. § 36-2201 to § 36-2208 (West Supp. 1999)
Ark. Code Ann. § 20-13-101 to § 20-13-707 (Supp. 1999)
Calif. Code Health & Safety § 1791 to § 1799.200 (West Supp. 1999)
Colo. Rev. Stat. § 25-3.5-101 to § 25-3.5-709 (Supp. 1999)
Conn. Gen. Stat. Ann. § 19a-175 to § 19a-196(b) (Supp. 1999)
Del. Code Ann. § 9701 to § 9706, § 9801 to § 9814 (Supp. 1999)
D.C. NO CODE SECTIONS (Supp. 1999)
Fla. Stat. Ann. § 401.01 to § 401.481 (West Supp. 1999)
Ga. Code Ann. § 31-11-1 to § 31-11-82 (Supp. 1999)
Hawaii Rev. Stat. § 321-221 to § 321-232, § 453-31 to 453-33 (personnel)
    (Supp. 1999)
Idaho Code § 39-139 to § 39-146A (West Supp. 1999)
Ill. Ann. Stat. Ch 210 § 50/2 to 50/33 (Smith Hurd Supp. 1999)
Ind. Code Ann. § 16-31-1-1 to § 16-31-10-2 (Burns Supp. 1999)
Iowa Code Ann. § 147A.1 to 147A.28 (West Supp. 1999)
Kan. Stat. Ann. § 65-6201 to § 65-6151 (Supp. 1999)
Ky. Rev. Stat. § 211.950 to § 211.968, §311.650 to 311.658 (paramedics),
    §411.148 (non-liability) (Supp 1999)
La. Rev. Stat. 40 § 1231 to 40 § 1236 (West Supp. 1999)
32 Maine Rev. Stat. Ann. § 81 to § 94 (Supp. 1999)
Md. Ann. Code § 13-501 to § 13-599, § 14-301 to § 14-305, § 4-601 to § 4-602
    (Supp 1999)
Mass. Gen. Laws Ann. 111C § 1 to § 15 (Michie/Law Co-Op Supp. 1999)
Mich. Comp. Law. Ann. § 333.20901 to § 333.20979 (Supp. 1999)
Minn. Stat. Ann. § 144E.001 to § 144E.52 (West Supp. 1999)
Mo. Ann. Stat. § 190.001 to § 190.500 (Vernon Supp. 1999)
Miss. Code Ann. § 41-59-1 to § 41-59-77, § 41-60-11 to 41-60-13 (Supp. 1999)
Mont. Code Ann. § 50-6-101 to § 50-6-506 (Supp. 1999)
Neb. Rev. Stat. § 71-5172 to § 71-51000 (Supp. 2000)
Nev. Rev. Stat. Ann. § 450B.010 to § 450B.900 (Supp. 1999)
NH Rev. Stat. Ann. § 151-B:1 to § 151-B:24 (Supp. 1999)
NM Stat. Ann. § 24-10A-1 to § 24-10B-12 (Supp. 1999)
NJ Stat. Ann. § 26:2K-1 to 26:2K-62 (West Supp. 1999)
NY Code. R. R. Title 10 § 800.1 to § 800.90 (Mckinney Supp. 1999)
NC Gen. Stat. § 143-507 to § 143-533 (EMS act), § 131E-155 to § 131E-161
    (ambulance services) (Supp. 1999)
ND Cent. Code § 23-27-01 to § 23-27-05 (Supp. 1999)
Ohio Rev. Code Ann. § 4765.01 to § 4765.99 (Supp. 1999)
Okla. Stat. Ann. Title 63 § 1-2501 to § 1-2516 (West Supp. 1999)
Or. Rev. Code § 682.015 to § 682.991 (Supp. 1999)
28 Pa. Cons. Stat. Ann § 1001.1 to § 1013.7 (Purdon Supp. 1999)
RI Gen. Laws. § 23-4.1-1 to § 23-4.1-15 (Supp. 1999)
SC Code Ann. § 44-61-10 to § 44-61-150 (Law Co-Op Supp. 1999)
SD Codified Laws § 34-11-1 to § 34-11-10, § 34-11A-1 to § 34-11A-33, § 36-4B-1 to
    § 36-4B-36 (Supp. 1999)
Tenn. Code Ann. § 68-140-101 to § 68-140-604 (Supp. 1999)
Tex. Code Ann. Health & Safety § 773.001 to § 773.148 (Vernon Supp. 1999)
Utah Code Ann. § 26-8-1 to § 26-8-15, § 26-8A-101 to § 26-8A-601 (Supp 1999)
Vt. Stat. Ann. CH 71 § 2651 to § 2688 (Supp. 1999)
Va. Code § 32.1-111.1 to § 32.1-116.3 (Supp. 1999)
Wash. Rev. Code. Ann. 18.73.005 to § 18.73.921 (Supp. 1999)
W. Va. Code Ann. § 16-4C-1 to § 16-4C-23 (Supp. 1999)
Wis. Stat. Ann. § 146.50 to § 146.59 (West Supp. 1999)
Wyo. Stat. Ann. § 33-36-101 to § 33-36-113 (Supp. 1999)

Source: Collected from the actual legislative materials for each jurisdiction by the author.
KEY § = section; Ann. = Annotated; Rev. = Revised; Stat. = Statutes; Supp. = Supplement

EMS and the Judicial System

Over the years, the EMS field has been relatively unscathed by major lawsuits in the judicial system. This trend may be attributable to several factors. First, EMS is a young profession. EMS has only been recognized as an occupation within the last thirty years. In addition, until recently, volunteers or technicians with little professional training provided the majority of EMS. Many modern EMS agencies lack appropriate financial resources and are government based. Therefore, lawsuits against volunteers or the government are traditionally unpopular and unsuccessful. Moreover, if the EMS agency does not have the financial resources to pay a settlement, collecting from an EMS agency may force the agency to close, thus disrupting or terminating EMS in that community. To help protect such EMS programs, most states have immunity statutes that severely limit the monetary damages that can be collected from an EMS-related lawsuit.

However, these days the public is better educated and more health care savvy. The media bombards citizens with television shows depicting "real life" trauma and emergencies. As a result of popular culture's dramatization of the EMS industry, expectations of EMS continue to grow. Technological advances have also changed the EMS provider's role, equipping EMTs with more high-tech tools and resources to use in their everyday efforts to save lives. Such technology is often falsely portrayed by the media as being fail-safe and always effective. When an ambulance does not arrive on the doorstep before the caller hangs up the phone, the media-saturated public is disappointed. When an EMS provider is unable to save a life, his or her position as a health care professional is questioned. Such disappointment in and questioning of EMS can sometimes lead to someone contacting a lawyer. At that point, it is easy for the EMS provider, the agency, and the system to be transformed from Good Samaritans to defendants.

Entering the Judicial System

The legal system was created to instill and promote a sense of justice and fairness. It is a forum in which disputes are resolved according to the laws, not an individual's social or economic standing, political beliefs, popularity, or other factors. The legal system strives toward the ideal of equality of treatment for all. In the past, EMS tended to have little interaction with the judicial system. Today, however, increased accountability checks by the public have caused EMS litigation to occur more frequently. It is likely that the average EMS provider will have at least one first-hand encounter with the courts during his or her career.

The United States judicial system has divided the courts into federal and state courts. A federal court hears matters pertaining to federal laws, cases that exist between parties from differing states, and those involving large sums of money. Federal criminal courts have jurisdiction over violations of federal criminal laws and some federal regulations that have criminal sanctions, such as some drug regulations. Federal civil courts have jurisdiction over cases involving large sums of money or cases involving individuals and entities from multiple states.

Legally Speaking

civil action A lawsuit brought by an individual (the plaintiff) against another individual, corporation, or entity (the defendant) seeking to redress (through monetary damages or other court orders) harm that the plaintiff suffered as a result of the defendant's actions.

criminal action A claim brought by the federal or state government on behalf of the citizens alleging a violation of the law that may result in the defendant being punished by fines, incarceration, or possibly the death penalty.

The state courts hear cases at different levels, depending on the location of the court, the nature of the case, and potential monetary value of the case. State criminal courts have jurisdiction over violations of state criminal laws. State civil courts have jurisdiction over most civil matters. Traffic violations are normally heard in municipal, or city, courts. Municipal courts also hear cases involving nominal monetary disputes or damages. Courts of general state jurisdiction are reserved for cases that do not rise to the federal level or contain federal questions of law, but may involve large sums of money. It is most likely that an EMS provider's court experience will occur in a state court of general jurisdiction. This is the court that normally hosts cases involving negligence and medical malpractice.

A **civil action** occurs when an individual (the plaintiff) initiates a lawsuit against a person, corporation, or entity (the defendant) because he or she suffered harm as a result of the defendant's actions. In a civil action suit, the plaintiff makes a tort claim in which he or she seeks redress (satisfaction or amends) from a defendant for an alleged act, damage, or injury (other than a broken contract). Redress is usually sought in the form of a monetary sum, but it may also be sought in the form of an administrative remedy such as an injunction or a "cease and desist" order. Examples of tort claim actions include an alleged negligent act, slander, libel, defamation, and acts that lead to personal injury. An EMS provider most commonly faces a lawsuit that involves negligence because a particular service or duty was not provided. There are four elements in every tort action involving negligence:

1. The existence of a legal duty for the defendant to service the plaintiff in a reasonable and competent manner;
2. Breach of that duty;
3. Proximate causation, or link, between the defendant's actions or inactions in breaching his or her legal duty and the resulting harm to the plaintiff;
4. Quantifiable damages incurred by the plaintiff as a result of the defendant's actions or inactions.

The elements of a negligence action are discussed in further detail in Chapter 7.

In a **criminal action,** the government brings legal action against a person who has been charged with violating a law. (For more information on criminal actions, see Chapter 9.) A criminal action is separate and distinct from any civil actions that may arise from the same event. In a civil action, the injured party, not the government, is suing the defendant for harm that was incurred. Criminal actions, on the other hand, are brought on by the federal or state government on behalf of the public and may result in various types of penalties, including monetary fines, incarceration, or even the death penalty, depending on the jurisdiction and the action(s) charged.

Within the criminal court system, there are two types of charges, a felony and a misdemeanor. The severity of the punishment for being found guilty depends on the type of crime. Usually a misdemeanor involves a fine and perhaps some jail time (usually less than one year).

A felony, on the other hand, usually involves **incarceration** for at least one year and may include financial penalties.

The Constitution prohibits an individual from being tried more than once in criminal court for the same offense. Being tried twice for the same crime is known as "double jeopardy." Suing someone civilly for monetary damages based on the same actions that result in criminal charges is not considered double jeopardy and is permissible under state and federal law. In order to be found guilty in a criminal matter, the government must convince a jury that the defendant is guilty of the crime charged *beyond a reasonable doubt.* The amount of certainty required to permit a juror to rule against a defendant is known as the "standard of proof." The standard of proof in a criminal action is much higher than the standard of proof in a civil action. The standard of proof in a civil action is usually based on the defendant being proven responsible *by a preponderance of the evidence presented,* which is a much less stringent burden of proof than criminal proceedings. Therefore, it is much easier for a plaintiff to prove a defendant liable in civil court than the government to prove a defendant guilty in criminal court.

To better understand how the government and EMS providers interact with each other, consider this example: An EMT responds to a caller who reports shortness of breath. While in transit, the EMT drives at an excessive speed through a busy intersection and collides with another motor vehicle, killing its driver. In this situation, a police officer may arrest the EMT for the felony crime of causing the other driver's death. It is likely that the EMT will be charged with a crime by the district attorney. A grand jury will hear the preliminary evidence and may indict the EMT for that charge. Based on the indictment, the EMT will have to stand trial in a criminal court. The goal of this proceeding will be to determine whether the EMT is guilty of causing the death of the other driver. If found guilty, the EMT may be subject to incarceration, financial penalties, probation, or a combination of these penalties.

Separate from the criminal proceeding, the estate of the deceased driver may file a civil lawsuit that seeks monetary damages from the EMT. In this proceeding, the case will be heard in a civil court. The goal of this proceeding will be to determine the EMT's liability for the wrongful death of the driver. Subsequent to this proceeding—regardless of the findings in the related criminal proceeding—the EMT may be liable for a financial judgment that he or she will have to pay to the estate of the deceased driver.

Determination of Damages

In deciding how best to proceed in a civil action, the plaintiff's attorney will evaluate the potential **damages** that the plaintiff may seek to recover. The plaintiff's attorney evaluates the injuries or wrongs sustained by his or her client and places a monetary value on these grievances.

Plaintiff damages are determined by several factors: the sex and age of the plaintiff, the plaintiff's occupation and remaining productive working years, the specific nature of the injuries, and the magnitude of the defendant's alleged actions. Typically, experts are called into the courtroom to testify about the injured party's economic future as it stood before the

Legally Speaking

incarceration The loss of certain personal rights, including freedom through commitment to a penal institution, as a result of being found guilty, by a court of competent jurisdiction, of committing a criminal offense.

damages Economic value of the harm caused to another; the loss, injury, or deterioration caused by negligence, design, or accident of one person to another in respect to the alleged victim's person or property; a monetary valuation of the loss sustained by the injured party.

Legally Speaking

compensatory damages The cost associated with the actual harm caused that correlates to returning the plaintiff to the same standard of living and quality of life that he or she experienced before the alleged harm.

gross negligence An act of negligence caused by actions that are willful, wanton, or a recklessly disregard of a required duty or standard.

punitive damages Compensation assessed in excess of actual damages as a form of punishment for willful and malicious civil conduct.

Legal Practices

An EMS provider may be found grossly negligent if it is proven that he or she knew or should have known that injuries or an aggravation of illness was likely to occur based upon his or her action or inaction. Gross negligence may also be found when an EMT intentionally inflicts an injury or aggravates an injury or illness.

incident and how the incident has affected the plaintiff's future earnings and overall financial well-being.

There are several types of damages. **Compensatory damages** are sought in all cases. These damages address the specific cost of the harm that occurred. The goal of compensatory damages is to return the injured individual to the same standard of living and quality of life that he or she experienced before the incident. Compensatory damages may include payment of medical bills and lost wages or compensation for pain and suffering.

Should the case be one of **gross negligence,** or an intentional act, where the court finds that the defendant purposely caused or intended to cause harm, the court on its own discretion may seek to award **punitive damages,** additional fees to effectively "punish" the party found liable. In certain extreme circumstances, the court may also award "treble" damages, or triple the monetary damages to be paid to the offended party. These additional damages are, typically, specific to the state and the type of tort involved in the case and are regulated by statute.

Here is an example of how the awarding of damages works:

A local EMS provider is found liable for gross negligence in responding recklessly to a call from a 45-year-old man with chest pain when it is proven in a court of law that the man died as a direct and proximate result of the negligence of the EMS department. The deceased was married with two young children. He was an engineer with a career expectancy of 20 more years and a life expectancy of 35 more years. During the trial, an economist testifies that the engineer had been earning $65,000 a year, and that based on increases in salary, benefit packages, retirement savings and investments the projected value of his natural life—had he not met his untimely death—would be valued at $2,974,528.00. In addition to awarding this sum for damages, the court may award about $200,000 for the pain and suffering of the deceased and his family.

Normally, total damages awarded would also compensate for the loss of marital relations on behalf of the wife, the loss of companionship on behalf of the children, as well as any additional income from side jobs or hobbies of the deceased that produced monetary gain for the family. A final verdict may award as much as $4 million to the family of the deceased.

Future Trends in EMS Litigation

As the public becomes better educated, and as the media continues to promote healthier lifestyles and "reality" trauma television and movies, it is anticipated that litigation against EMS providers will rise. Unfortunately, because EMS providers are a part of the health care industry, some plaintiffs see them as an easy target for civil liability. As EMS departments seek to function more like businesses by contracting services for special events, educational seminars, and nonemergency transports, this perception may rise. Further, health insurance companies are eager to be reimbursed by negligent parties for monies they pay out in claims, and EMS providers are likely to be the target of this form of restitution.

Because the EMS field is still a young occupation, it will likely encounter growing pains. Previously functioning by driving a hearse with a red light that delivered the patient to the hospital or directly to the funeral home, EMS providers now offer more advanced technologies in the field, such as 12-lead ECGs and immediate-acting, clot-dissolving pharmaceuticals. EMS providers also use helicopters and critical care transport ambulances to deliver patients to level 1 trauma centers. As technology becomes more advanced, EMS providers take on the greater responsibility for providing more thorough medical service to the community. With this additional responsibility comes additional accountability. Thus, the door opens to a greater likelihood of litigation.

Before the late 1980s, EMS litigation was almost nonexistent. When litigation did occur, it typically involved traffic violations rather than the negligent delivery of medical treatment. In the 1990s litigation increased, and because it is a lengthy process to resolve a lawsuit, it has only been within the last decade that significant verdicts have been rendered against EMS providers.

The trend for courts to rule against EMS providers can be discouraging for those who are trying to save lives. How and why is the trend moving away from the comfortable immunity that we previously experienced? How can we reverse this trend and continue to provide quality care to our communities? How do we protect our coworkers, our departments, and ourselves from time-consuming and financially draining litigation?

Recently, several court decisions have been handed down that sound the warning signal for future immunity provisions for the EMS profession. One particular case, *Staccia v. City of Columbus,* exemplifies this notion that EMS providers are to be held more accountable out in the field. Whereas the majority of the justices in this appeals court decision **held** that the EMS providers were not liable under a theory of immunity, there was a **dissenting** opinion. In his dissenting opinion, Justice Tayak suggests that EMS providers escape liability because there is an assumption that the harm caused in a negligent action must only be physical. Justice Tayak suggests that emotional harm should be considered as well as physical harm. As a result of this dissenting opinion, simply relying on EMS treatment protocols as a justification for going against a patient's wishes may not provide protection against liability in subsequent cases because doing so may cause emotional harm to the patient.

However, as discussed in Chapter 6, a majority of jurisdictions do continue to provide immunity for EMS providers. Accordingly, many cases are dismissed without making it to trial. This trend may change. In *Hire et al. v. Mayor and City Council of Baltimore et al.,* the District Court of the District of Maryland held "whether a defendant possesses a qualified immunity is ultimately an issue of law for the court to determine. . . . To the extent the issue hinges on factual disputes that must be resolved by the . . . jury, the Court will not resolve the issue on preliminary motion (before a trial)." In this statement, the scope of immunity for EMS providers is clearly being questioned by the courts and does not remain a luxury that will be guaranteed into the future.

Legal Practices

Keep in mind that the jury is responsible for determining the monetary value of damages given to the injured party. The jury is composed of ordinary, reasonable people. Anyone may be called to serve on a jury. However, the judge presiding over the case may ultimately limit or award additional damages depending on state and federal statutes as well as the nature and severity of the case.

Legally Speaking

holding The rule of law that comes from a case decision (also referred to as held or hold).

dissent An opinion that disagrees with the majority opinion and is not a rule of law.

Conclusion

As EMS develops and evolves from informal public services into a formal health care delivery service, the liability and accountability of EMS providers changes. It is vital to the future growth and development of the EMS provider that these changes in accountability and liability be understood and expected. Becoming familiar with legal principles and terminology will help EMS providers protect themselves.

You Be the Judge

Discussion

Although state statutes commonly guide the use of lights and sirens during an ambulance's response to rescue calls, they rarely dictate what speed is considered reckless. Therefore, the EMT must take full responsibility for driving decisions. In the situation presented at the beginning this chapter, it is likely that the EMT would be found to be guilty of a criminal charge (driving faster than the listed speed in a school zone during school hours, thus causing negligent vehicular homicide). The EMT would also likely be found liable in civil actions concerning the personal injury sustained by the student. In this example, who is on the jury may also affect the ruling. If the jury is composed of parents, a higher monetary award may be given to the family of the injured party. In addition, it is more likely that the jury will be persuaded to find the EMT guilty of excessive speed, even if the speed while responding was only 9 mph over the posted limit.

Bibliography

Hire et al. v. Mayor and City Council of Baltimore et al., United State District Court of the District of Maryland, MSG-952507 (1997).

Staccia v. City of Columbus, Ohio App. LEXIS 5852, (1994).

Chapter 2

Navigating Through a Lawsuit

You Be the Judge

You are at the fire station. A pizza delivery person arrives with three deluxe supreme pizzas and asks if you are Bob. You say, "Yes, I am," anticipating that you have been stuck with the bill for the food. In addition to the pizzas, you are handed a complaint. Being lawsuit savvy, you:

1. Immediately drop the legal paperwork to the ground, being careful to maintain your grip on dinner.

2. Hand the paperwork back to the delivery guy with his menial tip, stating you are not accepting the complaint.

3. Place the complaint in the trash, thinking you have done nothing wrong so you can ignore it.

4. Keep the document and contact your attorney and ask her to come to the station to review the complaint that you have been served.

Case Study

One night while working the overnight shift, you hear the tones sound.

"Attention Village Volunteer Fire Department, rescue is needed at 123 Park Place for a woman with difficulty breathing. Page out at 2:13 am."

Your sleep is shattered. You quickly dress as you race out of your front door to head down to the fire department. Shaking yourself awake you reach for a piece of gum to ward off morning breath, and mentally prepare for arrival at 123 Park Place. You hear the second page at 2:15 am. Moments later you arrive at the fire station, meeting two other EMTs at the door.

"Rescue 204 to Village."

"Go ahead 204."

Case Study, continued

"204 is en route to 123 Park Place with three EMTs."

"Village copies 204 en route to 123 Park Place with three EMTs at 2:17 am."

The snow is heavy, and the squad slides precariously as the wheels crunch through the freshly-blanketed streets. A bridge is out, and you navigate a detour toward 123 Park Place.

"204 to Village."

"Go ahead 204."

"204 is on scene."

"Village copies 204 on scene at 2:23 am."

You are inside the house in what you believe to be record time. Upon entering, you find a 38-year-old female, with a past medical history of asthma, in full cardiac arrest. You find the patient to be unresponsive, apneic, and pulseless. Immediately, you and your fellow EMTs perform basic life support by starting chest compressions and providing respirations with a bag-valve-mask device and oropharyngeal airway. Without your interventions, the patient's pulse and respiratory rate would remain at zero. While continuing your best efforts you load your patient into the rescue squad.

"204 to Village."

"This is Village, go ahead 204."

"204 is en route to Village Community Hospital and performing CPR."

"Village copies. 204 en route with CPR in progress to Village Community Hospital at 2:42 am."

You continue your efforts en route.

"204 to Village."

"This is Village, go ahead 204."

"204 is out at Village Community."

"Village copies 204 out at Village Community at 2:52 am."

The emergency department implements full advanced cardiac life support measures, but the patient is pronounced dead at 3:17 am. The deceased was a vice president of a major pharmaceutical company and mother of four young children. Her grieving husband is a partner in a prominent law firm.

You return to the station, reviewing the call over and over in your mind. You wonder if the deceased patient's husband will file a lawsuit against you and the department. As you mentally relive the 19 minutes you spent on the scene, you wonder if there was anything else you or your partners could have done in responding to this call.

The Anatomy of a Lawsuit

Whenever a client enters a law office, the attorney must carefully discern whether a **cause of action** exists before embarking on the filing of a lawsuit in court. In the case study described above, does a valid cause of action exist?

To determine the cause of action and the potential value of a case, an attorney typically interviews as many people as possible to gather appropriate information. In addition, the attorney may seek out expert opinions and request public records, such as police reports and 9-1-1 tapes, as well as private documents, such as **medical records** and human resources files.

In the case study presented, the first medical record to be obtained would most likely be the incident's run report, the standardized report that must be completed by EMS providers for each incident to which they respond. Based on federal and state privacy laws, such as the federal Healthcare Insurance Portability and Accountability Act (HIPAA), the attorney may have to follow certain procedures to gain access to these documents, such as issuing a subpoena or obtaining a court order. When such formalities are met, the attorney is able to examine the records and determine if a cause of action exists.

In this case study, the attorney will most likely engage a medical, nursing, or EMS expert consultant to review the run report and closely scrutinize the care rendered to determine if the appropriate **standard of care** was met and the appropriate **protocols** were followed. An expert is someone who has extensive education, training, and experience is his or her field. To be recognized as an expert witness by a court, the expert must submit a resume or curriculum vitae for scrutiny by the court and opposing counsel. The opposing attorney has the right to cross-examine an expert witness and challenge his or her credibility and competence before the court accepts the testimony. For example, an emergency physician who is on a medical school faculty, works in a busy trauma center, and has researched and published articles on the clinical aspects of prehospital care would be considered an expert in the clinical aspects of EMS.

In the case study presented, an attorney may argue that there is a possible claim of **negligence** against the EMTs and the Village Fire Department. Such a claim may stem from the long response time in arriving on scene, as well as the failure to provide more advanced care while en route to the hospital. Particularly, the attorney could question the failure of the squad personnel to intubate the trachea and give medications either via the endotracheal tube or through an intravenous line. In addition, no effort was made to defibrillate the patient.

Before actually filing a lawsuit, the attorney reviews the **statute of limitations.** In this case study, it is likely that the attorney would base the cause of action on the theory of negligence, which in most states carries with it a two- or three-year statute of limitations. This means that the injured party has two or three years from the time of the injury to file a lawsuit in the proper court. If the lawsuit is not filed within the requisite period, regardless of the injury or the wrongful actions of the provider, the injured party, or **plaintiff,** is barred from filing such a lawsuit. The attorney may also seek to file this case under the theory of medical malpractice, particularly against the medical control of Village Fire EMS. Medical malpractice is a type of negligence that specifically concerns the quality of medical care provided. In general, although this time frame varies state to state, a medical malpractice action must be brought within two years from the time in which the medical

Legally Speaking

cause of action The legal basis for a lawsuit.

medical record A document containing confidential personal information regarding the health status of a person; created by a health care provider during the provision of medical care.

standard of care The degree of care that a reasonably prudent provider of similar certification level should render under similar circumstances.

protocols Written instructions that dictate necessary actions to be taken under various specific circumstances, usually developed by regional medical control personnel and considered to be the standing medical orders for that region.

negligence Failure to exercise the degree of care to which a person of ordinary prudence (a reasonable person) would exercise under the same circumstances that results in injury or damage to another.

statute of limitations A period set by law that specifically limits the amount of time in which a lawsuit can be filed.

plaintiff The party who files a civil action for recovery of damages, claiming he or she has been harmed by the defendant.

Legal Practices

Statutes of limitations vary from state to state. EMS providers need to be fully aware of their state's limitations and time frames for filing lawsuits.

Legally Speaking

notice of intent A letter notifying the defendant of the future possibility of the filing of a lawsuit by the plaintiff, which in some states extends the statute of limitations for a specified length of time; some states also require such notice if filing a suit against a state agency.

defendant The party against whom relief or recovery is sought; the party must defend or deny a cause of action.

complaint The initial document of a lawsuit filed in a court that describes the plaintiff's claims against the defendant.

answer The defendant's written response to the plaintiff's filed complaint.

pleading Written documents filed in court that set forth the plaintiff's cause of action and the defendant's grounds of defense.

malpractice was discovered. Some states have additional prefiling requirements, such as review of the claim by a medical malpractice tribunal or commission consisting of legal and medical professionals. The filing of a **notice of intent** by a potential plaintiff or his or her attorney may extend this one-year time limit. The notice of intent essentially adds 6 months to the time limit required for the initial filing of the complaint in states that have this law.

It is most common for an EMS provider to be sued for negligence rather than medical malpractice because the EMS provider usually works under the medical control of the physician, meaning the EMS provider is simply following the practice protocols and instructions of the licensed physician. However, it is possible for an EMS provider to be named within a medical malpractice action, and thus be notified of a pending lawsuit within the one-year time frame.

If the statute of limitations of an incident runs out without an ensuing lawsuit, don't assume that you are free and clear of a legal battle. Be aware that there are certain exceptions to general statutes of limitations, such as the filing of a lawsuit on behalf of a minor. In some jurisdictions, a child who sustains an aggravation of injury or an illness may either have a lawsuit filed on his or her behalf by the legal guardian (known as a "next friend") or that child may wait to bring the lawsuit on his or her own behalf when of legal age. In such jurisdictions, a minor is permitted to wait until age 18 plus two additional years to file a negligence action. For example, an infant that is treated in a motor vehicle accident may be permitted to wait until he is 20 years old to file a negligence complaint against the EMS provider who cared for him.

In the case study presented earlier in the chapter, the lawsuit would be filed within one year of the patient's date of death. The deceased patient's survivors or the deceased estate would be the plaintiff bringing the action forward in civil court. The plaintiffs would seek amends for the perceived wrongful death of their loved one. The EMTs and the Village Fire Department would be named **defendants.**

To start the lawsuit process, the plaintiff's attorney files a document known as the **complaint.** The complaint enumerates specific actions believed to have been made by the defendants that directly caused the death of the patient. In the case study discussed in this chapter, the plaintiffs would probably view the EMTs as negligent, and base their case on the belief that their wife and mother would have survived her asthma attack if the EMTs had responded promptly and treated her condition appropriately.

Once a complaint is filed it must be answered by the defendant in a timely manner. Usually court rules require the filing of an **answer** within 28 days; however, an extension may sometimes be granted if the defendant petitions the court. Each written document filed with the court, including the complaint, answer, and various motions, is known as a **pleading.** The format of the pleadings as well as the timelines of filing the pleadings, are governed by the statutory "Rules of Civil Procedure" for that particular jurisdiction.

The EMTs and the Village Fire Department would presumably respond in a timely fashion, and deny the allegations of the plaintiffs. In addition, the defendants would respond with **affirmative defenses**—the reasons why they are not liable for the death of the patient, even if the facts as alleged by the plaintiffs are accurate. In most jurisdictions throughout the United States, the EMTs in this case study would be able to use **sovereign immunity** (immunity of the government or government-funded entities from certain civil suits) as a defense and could request the charges be dismissed before going to trial.

However, because private ambulance services rather than governmental agencies or departments employ many EMS providers, they are not protected by sovereign immunity. However, many jurisdictions have specific immunity statutes that limit the liability of emergency medical personnel. In some states, such immunity statutes, referred to as "Good Samaritan laws," protect anyone who renders emergency care in good faith. "Good faith" means that the defendant did not intend to cause any harm. His or her actions were performed without malice and were not grossly negligent. Other states limit such "Good Samaritan" laws to individuals who are not paid for their services. These states typically have other specific immunity statutes for professional EMS providers. For example, Massachusetts law states that *"No emergency medical technician certified . . . and no police officer or firefighter, who in the performance of his duties and in good faith renders emergency first aid or transportation to an injured person or to a person incapacitated by illness shall be personally in any way liable as a result of rendering such aid . . ."* (See M.G.L.A. 111C §21.) All EMS providers should check with their agency's legal counsel to learn the existing immunities within a specific jurisdiction.

The court system is subject to rules that are declared publicly by the legislature to ensure the effective administration of justice. For example, if this case study were filed in a federal court, based on the federal rule of civil procedure 12(b)(6), the defense, at that time, would be permitted to file a motion, commonly referred to as a 12(b)(6) motion to dismiss. In this motion, the defense would argue that even if all the facts alleged in the complaint are correct, the plaintiff has not stated a claim from which relief may be sought. If the judge agrees, the judge may dismiss the case on his or her own accord. If it is determined that the EMS providers responded in an appropriate time, followed their protocol exactly, and nothing else could have been reasonably done, and both sides agree to these facts, no breach of duty occurred and therefore there is not a valid claim. However, if there are disputes of fact or if the plaintiff's claim is still valid, the case will move forward.

After a complaint has been filed and answered, and motions by the defendant to dismiss have been denied by the court, the case moves toward the **discovery** stage. Discovery is the process by which all available information requested regarding the case is exchanged between sides. Only information that is requested is provided; however, all information that is requested must be produced. Information may be obtained through document requests, written questioning, or interviews. Typically, one side of the case has various documents that are important to all sides of the case.

In the case study we are discussing, a supervisor of the EMTs may have conducted a routine follow-up investigation into the call in question. The supervisor's findings may have been compiled into a report and stored

---

Legally Speaking

affirmative defense A defense that is raised in the answer that, despite the truth of the facts of the complaint, excuses the defendant from liability; common examples of affirmative defenses include assumption of risk, contributory negligence, and self-defense.

sovereign immunity Doctrine that limits liability of state and local government entities; based on the old English common law theory that one cannot sue the king (ie, government).

discovery A phase of the civil action in which each side has an opportunity to gather relevant information associated with the case from the opposing side .

Legally Speaking

interrogatories Written questions from one party to another that must be answered in the discovery process.

deposition A discovery tool wherein factual and expert witnesses answer questions under oath in the presence of the respective attorneys; the testimony is recorded by audio, video, or a stenographer.

within the department's files. Without a formal request, the plaintiffs may never know about the report. However, once formally requested, the defendants must provide the report, along with any other documents pertaining to the call. Such a request may be specific or general. For example, the plaintiffs may request "all written documents in the custody of the department pertaining in any way to this call." Failure to provide the plaintiffs with the report may be a violation of civil procedure and may subject the department to fines and contempt charges. Only certain quality assurance documents, medical records, and personnel documents regulated by statutory privilege may be excluded from the discover process. The presiding court determines requests for such inclusion or exclusion. For example, documents that were prepared by a department's legal counsel may be considered privileged under principles of attorney-client confidentiality.

Legal Practices

Certain documents created in meetings related to peer review or quality assurance discussions may be privileged under state law. The law offers this protection because it is understood that there is educational value in reviewing previous rescue calls. Reviewing runs during quality assurance meetings gives the EMS provider an opportunity to effectively learn new tricks of the trade or fine-tune how new procedures are implemented. Learning is encouraged by the legislature, and thus this means of improving medical procedures and protocols is protected from exposure during a lawsuit. Quality assurance documents should not be stored with documents that are considered discoverable.

Keep in mind that even though some documents may be required to be given to opposing counsel, the court may not allow them to be introduced into evidence, meaning that the documents will not be seen by the jury, and therefore may not be considered by the jury when they make decisions regarding the outcome of a particular issue in the case. Check with your facility or municipal legal counsel to determine what documents are considered privileged in your jurisdiction.

Written questions, known as **interrogatories,** may be asked and answered by all parties involved in the litigation. Each attorney has the opportunity to send out a list of questions that must be answered by the opposing party within a certain period. Once the written answers have been received and documents have been forwarded to the appropriate attorney, those attorneys who submitted written questions may proceed with verbal questioning.

The pretrial process of verbally questioning a witness is known as a **deposition.** A deposition is one of the most important tools used by attorneys in the preparation for trial because it allows the attorneys for both sides to seek out facts and circumstances of which the witness has firsthand knowledge. A deposition also gives both sides of a case a chance to know whom the other side will be using for expert and factual witnesses.

In this chapter's case study, it is likely that each and every EMT that was on the scene during the incident in question would be deposed. In addition, the chief of the fire department, the dispatcher on duty, and the medical director may be deposed. The attorneys would also arrange depositions of expert witnesses. It is also likely that other defendants would be named in this lawsuit, such as the emergency physician on duty, the nursing staff present at the cardiac arrest, and perhaps even the family physician if the deceased patient recently received medical treatment.

A lot of information is learned at deposition. In this case study, the plaintiff's counsel may learn that volunteers—not permanent in-station, on-duty personnel—staff the department. The plaintiff's counsel may also learn that the easiest access road to 123 Park Place from the fire department was blocked because a bridge was out. Information regarding the current standards of education for EMTs as well as the standard of care that a basic EMT is qualified to deliver would also most likely be obtained. In this particular case study, the plaintiff's attorney may be under the impression that basic EMTs are qualified to orally intubate, start intravenous lines, and administer medications—skills that are actually reserved for higher-level paramedics.

With the knowledge learned from the deposition, the plaintiff's attorney would not be able to continue with the case against the EMS personnel and the fire department because it is likely that a jury would not find the EMTs negligent in their delivery of care because they performed their duties to the extent that their level of training and certification allowed. The attorney would not have discovered this pertinent information if the pretrial process of seeking expert opinions, preparing interrogatories, and deposing witnesses had not been followed. However, this case could continue against the personal physician of the deceased if the attorney discovers, for example, that the deceased had experienced adverse effects from a new medication.

If a case is viable enough to go forward after the depositions are finished, the attorneys must gear up for the next phase. Cases may be resolved via **mediation, arbitration, settlement,** or as a last resort, **trial.** For mediation and arbitration, a preliminary court appearance may be required to establish parameters, but the bulk of the matter is handled outside of court. For settlement and trials, court appearances are necessary for scheduling and the defining and limiting of issues specific to the case. The plaintiff's counsel and the defendant's counsel may write motions and briefs to limit or allow various pieces of evidence or testimony into the proceeding. Arguments for or against these requests may be made before the judge. A settlement conference may take place if a possibility for settling a case exists. At this time, a motion for **summary judgment** may be filed. This motion argues that the facts in dispute can only be viewed in one manner, and thus a full jury trial is not necessary to resolve the issue; the judge can decide the outcome of the case based on known case law.

Each participant in a trial has a specific role. The judge's role is to govern the proceedings and decide all issues of law. The jury is responsible for determining whether the defendant is responsible for any wrongdoing by reviewing the facts of the case that are in dispute. In essence, the jury applies an "ordinary reasonable person standard," meaning the jury asks the question: What would an average, ordinary, reasonable person do under similar circumstances? Sometimes the defendant waives a jury proceeding and no jury is used. In such circumstances, only the judge hears the case. This is known as a bench trial.

For the sake of saving time during a trial, the attorneys may choose to agree on certain facts of the case. For example, in this chapter's case study, the parties may agree or stipulate that it was snowing outside at the

---

Legally Speaking

mediation A process other than a trial in which the defendant and plaintiff actively participate in attempting to reach an agreement to a dispute; the proceedings are mediated by a neutral party.

arbitration The presentation of a disagreement to an impartial person or panel (agreed to by both parties) in a forum other than court, with the understanding that the decision reached by such arbitrator or arbitration panel is final.

settlement A private agreement between the parties that resolves the lawsuit without judicial intervention.

trial A formal proceeding governed by judicial oversight that resolves a conflict between two parties.

summary judgment Pretrial or preverdict judgment rendered by the court in response to a motion by the plaintiff or defendant, who claims that the absence of factual dispute on one or more issues eliminates the need to proceed with the trial or send those issues to the jury.

time of the call, and that the ground was covered with 4.5 inches of freshly fallen snow. With this stipulation in place, the jury would not have to hear evidence to determine whether it was snowing as the EMTs made their way to 123 Park Place; it would simply be understood.

Under a **dismissal without prejudice,** the party filing the lawsuit agrees to dismiss the lawsuit with the legal protection that the case may be refiled against the same parties, and on the same issues, within one year. This effectively adds an additional year to the statute of limitations, and allows the plaintiff's counsel extra time in seeking out pertinent information to assist their case at trial. If a case is **dismissed with prejudice,** the case cannot be litigated again, and the claim is dead.

Even if a case is not dismissed, it may be settled out of court for various reasons. Ninety percent of all cases are settled outside of the courtroom. Some cases are settled at a point during the trial itself. Settlements are commonly used to make a case "go away." Usually, a case is settled if it is deemed likely that the jury will award a large sum of money, or if there is fear regarding the potential negative publicity that may result from a trial. The insurance company representing the defendant commonly encourages settlements if they determine that the cost of pursuing a trial is significant or the probability of losing the case is high.

The term "nuisance value claims" refers to claims in which a defendant settles, even though the plaintiff does not have a strong case, because settlement is less expensive than litigating the claim. Just because a case is settled on behalf of the plaintiff does not necessarily indicate that the defendant was liable. Today, however, fewer cases are settled in this manner because insurance carriers are becoming more stringent in detecting and preventing insurance abuse and fraud.

If a case is not dismissed or settled, it proceeds to trial. All attorneys file trial briefs and prepare witnesses for trial. A jury is selected by means of **voir dire,** a process wherein the respective attorneys ask potential jury members a series of questions and are permitted to include or exclude a certain number from sitting on the jury. Through such questioning, the attorneys seek to include individuals sympathetic to their cause on the jury and exclude those who would not be sympathetic. After a jury has been selected, the trial may begin.

Trials may last for hours, months, or even years, depending on the complexity of the case. Each side has an opportunity to present an opening argument (a quick summation of the case) and witnesses, including experts, to explain the argument. Generally, witnesses are examined, or questioned, directly by the plaintiff's attorney. The defense attorney then has an opportunity to cross-examine each witness. The plaintiff's attorney always begins the trial. He or she must show the court that a cause of action exists.

After the plaintiff presents the case, the defendant has an opportunity to make a motion for a **directed verdict.** A directed verdict is a request by the defendant to dismiss the case in favor of the defense, claiming the plaintiff's attorney has failed to meet all of the requirements for a valid cause of action. If the judge agrees with the motion for directed verdict, the case is dismissed. If the judge determines that the plaintiff's attorney presented enough evidence to effectively support the cause of action at issue, he or she can refuse to grant the directed verdict, and the case continues. The defendant's attorney must then refute the allegations

Legally Speaking

dismissal without prejudice A dismissal of a claim on the grounds that it can be refiled within one year.

dismissal with prejudice A dismissal of a claim that is final and prevents the matter from being redressed in the future.

voir dire The process by which a jury is selected.

directed verdict A request by the defendant to dismiss the case in favor of the defense on the basis that the plaintiff's attorney failed to meet all of the requirements for a valid cause of action.

presented, set forth and support defenses, or present excusable justification for the defendant's actions.

After the defendant's viewpoint is presented via evidence and witnesses, the attorneys representing each party of the lawsuit prepare and present closing arguments. These arguments summarize the case made to the jury and attempt to influence the jury's review of the evidence presented during the trial.

After the closing arguments, the jury is given instructions by the judge. These instructions guide the jury in regards to which questions it is responsible for answering. Then the jury deliberations begin. Typically, these deliberations last only hours. It is rare for a civil jury to be sequestered (forced to stay isolated) while determining a verdict.

If the defendant is found liable, the jury then determines damages. Generally, a sympathetic jury awards higher monetary damages. Sometimes, the jury awards monetary damages that are too excessive to be considered just. In these situations, if the judge decides that the award far exceeds the extent of the liability, a judgment notwithstanding the verdict (JNOV) may be issued. A JNOV allows the judge to decrease the monetary damage award granted by the jury to the injured party based on the circumstances of the case and applicable laws.

The end of the trial rarely means that the case is over. Each side has an opportunity to appeal the decision of the judge or the jury. Such appeals must be made within a limited time frame (determined by the rules of the governing court) and must set forth a specific legal reason why the case must be reheard. It is not enough for a party to cry, "It's just not fair."

How could the Village Fire Department have been in the best position to defend or dismiss this lawsuit? Proper documentation is always the first step. Had the EMTs documented the adverse weather conditions and the need for a detour on the incident run sheet, it is likely that the plaintiff's counsel would have recognized that there was not an unreasonable delay in responding to the scene. Furthermore, the EMTs should have noted in their narrative the level of care provided and that such care was within their scope of certification and consistent with the guidelines of their local medical control protocol. Accurate and adequate documentation is not a guarantee against potential lawsuits, but it certainly assists in decreasing the risk of becoming a potential defendant.

What to Do If You Are Named in a Lawsuit

Anyone can sue anyone at anytime. Even if you perform your duties "by the book," you should never ignore the possibility that you will be sued.

If you are named as a party to a lawsuit, you will need a lawyer. Lawyers are trained in the rules of civil procedure and know the various legal nuances that complicate the simplified anatomy of the lawsuit presented in this chapter. As a defendant in a civil suit you will need to be represented by a civil defense attorney, preferably one with some EMS knowledge. Even if you are formally identified as just a witness in a legal proceeding, you should always be aware of your rights and potential liability. Your first step upon being formally notified of a pending legal action—whether the suit is filed against you, the department, or you and the department—is to notify your facility's administration and legal counsel. In most instances, the department will provide you with defense counsel. However, it must be noted that there may be situations in which your legal interests may conflict with the department's legal interests. If you belong to a union or EMS organization, you should check to see if membership entitles you to personal legal representation.

Defense attorneys are normally paid on an hourly basis. Their rates can vary. In addition to cost, you will need to keep several other factors in mind when selecting your attorney. For example, the department attorney may not have your best interests in mind if he or she is representing you *and* the department in the lawsuit. This is because the department's interests and your interests may not be identical. This situation may lead to inadequate representation on your behalf. You may wish to use as your defense the fact that you were provided with faulty equipment or inadequate training for the equipment you use. Your department, on the other hand, would want to deny the presence of faulty equipment to prevent bad publicity and departmental liability for inadequate training and upkeep of equipment. The potential conflicts, however, should not deter you from immediately notifying your department when served with legal notice. Failure to respond in a timely, appropriate manner to any filings may result in added liability and penalties to you and your department.

Initially, your attorney will ask you a barrage of questions about the events in question. It is in your best interest to be as truthful with the attorney as possible. Just as a patient who repeatedly denies taking any medications while being transported in the ambulance, and then offers an extensive list of medications to the emergency department nurse, interferes with your ability to do your job, hiding facts from your attorney can be detrimental to your case. Let your attorney judge whether a fact may be harmful. Everything that you tell the attorney will be kept confidential through the attorney-client privilege. In addition, unless your attorney has a background as an EMT or paramedic, you will probably have a greater EMS knowledge base than he or she will. Providing your lawyer with factual information, such as what really happened on the call, and copies of the EMS run reports, protocols, and regulations, may increase his or her knowledge and prevent surprises that may be revealed in discovery or trial.

You may also be deposed. As you prepare for your deposition, your attorney will discuss with you the types of questions that opposing counsel is likely to ask. Although your attorney will be with you throughout the deposition, only you will be able to answer the question. Your attorney will be permitted to object to questions or instruct you not to answer certain questions posed by the opposing counsel.

A deposition proceeding is generally much less formal than a trial. It is typically held at the office of your attorney or at the office of opposing counsel. Depositions vary in length according to the nature of the claim and your involvement. Be sure to schedule enough time for the deposition and advise your attorney of any physical conditions you may have that would require frequent breaks.

These points will help you prepare for your deposition and time on the witness stand at trial:

1. Always tell the truth, even if you believe it may hurt your case. Remember that you are under oath. Lying under oath is considered perjury, subject to punishment through criminal sanctions.

2. Wear neat, clean, comfortable attire. Your deposition may be videotaped and shown at trial, and your appearance portrays your credibility.

3. Listen carefully to the question being asked. If you do not understand the question, ask the attorney to repeat or rephrase the question.

4. Answer only the question being asked. Do not volunteer additional information.

5. Do not guess at the answer; if you do not remember, say that you do not remember.

6. You may be asked to review a document during a deposition. Thoroughly examine the document and think about the question before you answer.

7. Never volunteer to provide additional evidence.

8. Try to avoid saying "never" or "always."

9. Never express anger or start to argue with opposing counsel.

10. Try to minimize conversing with your attorney during the deposition.

Conclusion

Being sued can be a scary and stressful event, but EMS providers cannot be oblivious to the possibility of facing legal action. Understanding the process, and particularly your role in the process, will help reduce the stress that you may experience.

You Be the Judge

Discussion

Under Rules of Civil Procedure, a complaint is considered served and must be answered when (1) it is personally delivered to the correct party and (2) the correct party has physical receipt of the complaint by certified mail or hand-delivery. In the scenario presented at the beginning of the chapter, the correct action would be to contact your agency or attorney immediately. If you ignore the complaint, you can be found in contempt of court or guilty by default. If you are guilty by default, a court can issue a verdict against you and your agency. If you are not present in court and it is determined that you were properly notified, you are still obligated to pay whatever damages the jury determines are to be awarded. If you hand the complaint back to the server, you will probably still be considered to have been properly notified. Professional summons and complaint servers are trained to testify in court about how they attempted to deliver the complaint. If you refuse to accept a court order, you may be found in contempt of court in addition to defaulting. Contempt charges may lead to fines or incarceration.

Duties of the Legal System

You Be the Judge

While transporting a patient from a nursing home to the hospital, you and your partner drive by the scene of a two-car accident. Your patient is alert and conscious, but complains of a terrible headache. Her words are garbled and she is hard to understand. You attribute her condition to her age and do not believe she is suffering from any acute ailment. You stop at the scene of the accident, begin triage, call for help, and initiate patient care for three patients, none of whom are critically ill. Twenty-two minutes later, additional help arrives on scene. When you return to your original patient, you notice that she now has severe facial drooping and paralysis of her left side. What is your liability to the nursing home patient? Did you breach a duty of care? If so, what was that duty?

EMS providers enter the field with high ideals to serve the public, save lives, and reach out to individuals and families in their time of need when injury or illness strikes. They intend to assist the community in responding to day-to-day emergencies and disaster relief. EMS providers are also motivated to enter the field because they can be on the cutting edge of medicine. Moreover, EMS providers enter the field to become part of their community's public safety forces, helping to save lives and protect property. Whereas all EMS providers share these inspirations, goals, desires, and hopes, many of their responsibilities and duties are much more mundane.

The ABCs of EMS

Similar to the medical ABCs of EMS that all EMS providers are taught, in which the top priorities of patient care are always **A**irway, **B**reathing, and **C**irculation, the legal ABCs should be your top priorities when addressing your overall role as an EMS provider. Strict adherence to these three directives will help to ensure that you are compliant with your legally mandated duties as an EMS provider.

The Legal ABCs of EMS

The legal **ABCs** are:

ALWAYS DOCUMENT: Good documentation is essential. Most trials occur years after an event takes place. It is impossible to defend yourself against charges of wrongdoing if you must rely on your memory and speculation. A good rule of thumb to follow is, "if you did not document it, you did not do it." Therefore, always document your actions with the assumption that you will have to rely on such documentation several years later to defend yourself in a lawsuit. Make sure that you adequately document that all of your actions were within protocol. If your actions were not within protocol, explain why.

BE KIND TO YOUR PATIENT: You must treat every patient with respect and dignity. Always provide the best, most appropriate level of care that you are trained and certified to perform. In addition to being morally, ethically, and professionally required to do so, if you mistreat a patient, you will not be able to adequately defend your actions in a court of law.

CONTACT MEDICAL CONTROL: EMTs work under the authority of the medical license of the medical director or medical control physician. If there is ever any reason to deviate from established procedures or protocols or if there is a question regarding the clinical course of treatment, contact the medical control physician. Consulting with the medical control physician not only helps you to provide the best and most adequate patient care, it helps keep you out of legal trouble by showing that you consulted and followed the recommendations of the highest medical authority available.

> **Legally Speaking**
>
> **duty** A legally sanctioned obligation to perform a course of action originating from statutes, regulations, protocols, standards, policies, or case laws; if breached, the individual is liable.

Duty

The term **duty** is a legal term that refers to the actions that you are legally required to perform. By knowing and defining their duties, EMTs are able to effectively provide care and treat patients, as well as protect themselves and their coworkers from threatened litigation.

Duty to Self

The patient is often perceived as the most important part of the EMS call, but this is not necessarily true. Without the EMS provider rendering care, the patient would be no better off than before the call was dispatched. You have an ethical and legal duty to yourself to ensure that you can function in a proper and effective manner. This duty to self includes these actions:

1. *Duty to ensure proper accreditation.* You must be recognized to practice as an EMS provider in the jurisdiction where you work. Without proper accreditation through certification or licensure, you can be cited for practicing medicine without a license—a criminal offense. Make sure that all of your required accreditations are valid and up-to-date. You should also stay informed on any changes that may influence your accreditation. In many jurisdictions, your accreditation depends on the approval of a local medical director. Check with your medical director that you are in

Legal Practices

An EMT is faced with legal and ethical duties that facilitate the delivery of quality patient care. By upholding your ethical duties and maintaining clinical proficiency, you will fulfill most of the responsibilities involved in your legal duties.

good standing. Talk to your medical director. Get to know your medical director. You and your patients can benefit from a strong professional relationship that you develop with him or her.

2. *Duty to maintain your skills.* You have an obligation to remain proficient in all areas of care for which you are responsible. Using continuing education seminars, journals, research, and practice, you can ensure that your skills remain strong. If you feel that you are not as proficient in an area as you should be, you have a duty to review that material. Scheduling clinical rotations with specific departments in a hospital may help you maintain your proficiency.

3. *Duty to maintain your mental well-being.* EMS can be a highly stressful occupation. Without the proper interventions, you can become a victim of burnout. Even the best provider's ability to provide care can be destroyed by burnout. Talking amongst your peers about stressful calls, participating in Critical Incident Stress Debriefing sessions (consultations with trained stress and grief counselors to help you deal emotionally with posttraumatic stress), having a life outside the station, and doing something that is relaxing or enjoyable on a regular basis are all methods of caring for your mental needs. If you are off duty from work at a full-time EMS agency, you have no duty to respond unless you are on call, you specifically state at the incident that you are an EMS provider who can help, or you have already started to render assistance. The key thing to remember is: Do not make EMS your life 100% of the time. For more information check out *Managing Stress in Emergency Medical Services,* a part of this continuing education series.

4. *Duty to maintain your physical well-being.* Not being physically prepared to carry out your job responsibilities can place your patient in harm's way and create significant liability. The last thing that you want is a lawsuit that results from you dropping a patient down a flight of stairs. Further, a work-related injury could halt even the most promising career. Create and follow an exercise regimen, attempt to maintain a healthy diet, and avoid substance abuse of any kind. You have an absolute duty to not partake in any illicit substance while you are working. If you are involved in a work-related accident or incident and you are found to have been under the influence of an illicit substance while on duty, you will be held fully responsible for any damages that may have occurred.

Duty to Partner

Your second most important responsibility is to ensure the well-being of your partner. Whereas the global health care industry is just now becoming a team system, EMS has always been a team delivery system. Without your partner, you cannot effectively care for your patient.

You have a responsibility to ensure that your partner is healthy and capable of performing his or her duties at the beginning of every shift. If your partner is sick or injured, your ability to provide care is hindered. You have a duty to develop a working relationship with him or her in order to be able to best provide care for your patients. If you are aware of any issue that may hinder your partner's safe operation of a vehicle or adequate delivery of patient care, you have a legal duty to report or attempt to resolve such issues.

Duty of Responsibility for Equipment

Without properly functioning equipment, you cannot appropriately care for your patients within your scope of practice. If the defibrillator does not work or the batteries are not charged, your rapid response, your recent defibrillation update class, and your partner's well-being are irrelevant.

You are responsible for your equipment. You have a legal duty to check the status of your equipment at the beginning of each shift. If a piece of equipment is broken, you have an obligation to replace it. You will not do very well on the witness stand if the plaintiff's attorney asks you why you did not intubate a patient and your only answer is to blame the stock room technician for failing to put an airway kit on your unit before you left the station.

Duty to Patient

After you have accounted for yourself, your partner, and your equipment, you must focus on your responsibility to your patient. Respect the rights of the patient at all times. This means you must really listen to what the patient is and is not saying. This also means you should not talk down to a patient because they are poor, dirty, abusing a chemical substance, or from the "wrong part of town."

First, do no harm. It is your primary responsibility to ensure that none of your actions intentionally or accidentally cause physical or emotional harm to your patient. It is your duty to use your education and experience and effectively use the resources available to you at all times. This duty applies to all EMS providers, from the senior medic on the scene to the emergency department physician who is functioning as medical control. Doing no harm is not only limited to direct patient care, but encompasses all aspects of the emergency medical system. Failing to be aware of available resources or familiar with a new piece of equipment may be akin to not providing any aid at all.

Legal Practices

EMS providers become accustomed to the adrenaline rush of responding to emergencies and can develop a comfort level with distressful surroundings. Whereas a layperson may prefer to never set foot in an emergency department, for EMS providers it is a second home. Remember that an EMS provider's comfort zone is not the same as a patient's comfort zone, so you need to remain sensitive to the surroundings and emotional disposition of your patient. Situations that have become routine for you are usually distressing crises for your patients and their loved ones. Also, don't assume that, just because a patient is someone who regularly seeks EMS help, he or she doesn't have legitimate medical issues. You have a duty to treat every patient with the highest appropriate level of care.

You have a *duty to protect and honor the rights of your patient*. Every patient is granted specific and general rights under the United States Constitution, federal laws, state laws, and case law that have evolved from past lawsuits.

Violating the patient's rights is considered a violation of the "do no harm" duty. (See Chapter 4 for more information on patient's rights.)

An example of a patient right is the right to request or refuse medical treatment. Usually, the initial request for treatment comes in the form of a 9-1-1 call. Whether placed by the patient, a family member, or a by-stander, the call initiates an EMS response. Once the EMS team is on the scene, the patient may verbally ask for help. The patient may make a specific request for treatment by saying something such as, "Please help me stop my hand from bleeding. I cut myself with a knife," or the patient may just hold out the hand for immediate treatment.

A patient may request an EMS provider to stop medical treatment when the patient is not fully aware of the ramifications of the refusal or because he or she is unfamiliar or afraid of the procedure. Some patients may refuse treatment because they are apprehensive about the needles and pain involved in receiving injections or intravenous lines. Some patients may refuse treatment because they are embarrassed. In some cases, a patient may consent to treatment but not to be transported to the hospital, or he or she may only consent to transport, and then refuse treatment, such as an intravenous line or oxygen, en route because he or she is claustrophobic.

You also have the *duty to provide complete care to the patient*. It is your duty to alleviate as many of your patient's concerns as possible and to take the time to discover the source of the patient's discomfort. To perform this duty, you may need to explain every procedure that you anticipate providing to the patient as you travel to the hospital in easy-to-understand language or in great detail. Such a detailed explanation may be required in order for you to obtain a conscious and alert patient's informed consent or refusal of treatment.

In providing complete care to the patient, remember to treat the person as a whole. Considering the emotional consequences of illness and injury allows greater insight into total patient treatment. Sometimes, the signs or symptoms of a patient may be psychologically based. The patient's condition may also be affected by the physical surroundings of the scene or the people present during the patient's evaluation.

Providing complete care also involves maintaining a good attitude toward the patient and the health care system. Poor attitudes easily influence your ability (or perceived ability) to care for patients and may cause them increased anxiety if, for example, you refer to the patient's physician or receiving hospital in a negative way. In addition, if you belittle other health care providers, and your comments are proven inaccurate, you may suffer legal consequences in the form of a defamation action against you and your department. It is your duty to remain professional and truthful and to instill confidence in the treatment you are providing and the continuing care that the patient will receive upon entering the emergency department. By acting professionally and in the best interests of patients at all times, you can deliver the highest quality of care within your power.

In addition to treating physical injury or illness, EMS providers must also address a patient's emotional conditions. Individuals and their families are less likely to enter litigation for mistreatment if EMS personnel are respectful and address a patient's emotional issues. Addressing individuals as "Mister" or "Miss," "Sir" or "Ma'am" conveys respect and may facilitate a more meaningful exchange between you and the patient. Speaking calmly and communicating in a manner that is easily understood is imperative and leads to cooperation from the patient. If English is a patient's second language, try to communicate in the patient's primary language, if possible. In addition, respect the patient's privacy. For example, discreetly placing the leads for a 12-lead ECG may improve your rapport with the patient as well as limit the likelihood of violating the patient's rights.

Our duties do not end when the patient is delivered to the emergency department. The EMS provider still has a *duty to protect the privacy and confidentiality of the patient's medical history and records.* (See Chapter 11 for more information about documentation.) After the documentation process is completed, the medical run reports are kept in a secure place within the EMS agency. They are not subject to review by the general public. Medical run reports are separate from the documentation regarding EMS system operations. Operations documents, containing information such as the number of calls received in a specific time frame and the nature of those calls, may qualify as public records and are subject to public disclosure.

Private medical information regarding a patient's identity, diagnosis, or treatment is legally protected information. Release of such information without proper consent may be considered a violation of the patient's civil rights. Release of private medical information is governed by many federal and state laws, regulations, and case law. If you must release an EMS run report, your department should have a procedure regarding the request for release of such information. In certain instances, release forms must be signed by the patient or the patient's legal representative before a medical run record can be distributed or copied. *Never release a copy of an EMS run report or other patient information without first checking with your facility's administration or legal counsel.* This will ensure that proper policies and procedures for release of such protected information are followed.

Legal Practices

- Remember that it is sometimes necessary to "treat" the family of the patient. If possible, try to address the emotional needs of your patient's family. Emotional trauma that escalates often manifests itself physically in the form of symptoms, such as hyperventilation, fainting, or violently acting out. Additionally, the way you treat a loved one on the scene may affect that person's long-term emotional well-being as well as how they remember and reflect back on the traumatic event to which you were called.
- The patient is at his or her most vulnerable state when ill or injured.
- The rescue squad and emergency department are new, unfamiliar, cold, and sometimes scary places. We are familiar with these settings, and sometimes forget that it can be an unsettling experience for the patient.

Most departments use run reviews for quality assurance and improvement and educational purposes. Run reviews are held in accordance with stringent internal proceedings and should never be open to the public. Confidentiality must be protected. Keep in mind that a discussion of your latest, greatest rescue at the local bar may result in a lawsuit against you and the EMS agency for the improper disclosure of confidential and protected medical information.

Conclusion

As an accredited EMS provider, you are required to perform certain actions. These mandated actions are known as duties. Knowing your duties as an EMS provider is the first step in protecting yourself from unwanted legal action. Although the duties presented in this chapter may seem burdensome, they may actually be integrated into your job already. You have probably been performing these actions without realizing that they were mandated parts of your job. Conscious recognition of these duties, however, can assist you in providing the best care possible to your patients.

You Be the Judge

Discussion

Once patient care has been established, the EMS provider has an absolute duty to continue care of that patient until the patient is turned over to a provider of equal or higher certification. Failure to continue adequate care for a patient that you started to treat is known as *abandonment*. (See Chapter 8.) Although you may have a duty to stop and render aid at an accident scene that occurs within your service area, your primary duty is to the patient you are already treating. In the situation outlined at the beginning of this chapter, it was a bad idea for you to stop at the accident scene and then leave your original patient alone to treat those injured at the accident. Leaving the patient alone breaches your duty of providing continuous adequate care.

Severe headache, garbling of words, and difficulty communicating are all signs of a cerebrovascular accident (CVA) or stroke. As an EMT, it is your duty to be familiar with the signs and symptoms of a CVA and treat such presenting signs and symptoms appropriately. Attributing the patient's condition to her age and assuming she was not suffering from an acute ailment breaches the EMS provider's duty to properly assess and treat your patient. At a bare minimum, you should have assessed vital signs, obtained a medical history, probably administered oxygen, and continued to monitor the patient's condition and vital signs during the remainder of the transport.

The policies, procedures, protocols, and case law of the particular jurisdiction within which you practice determine whether you had a duty to stop at the accident. In most jurisdictions, if you already have a patient on board, radioing ahead to dispatch requesting additional units to the accident would fulfill your duty to assist. Otherwise, the delay in transport of the original patient caused by stopping to treat the new patients may prove detrimental to the original patient's condition. However, the law is clear in every jurisdiction that even if it is deemed appropriate to stop, only one provider should check on the accident victims. Someone of the same training or higher than you should always stay with the original patient.

In this case study scenario, you abandoned your patient, clearly breaching your duty of providing continuous adequate care. You would have an extremely difficult time defending your actions in court.

Chapter 4

Patient Rights

You Be the Judge

At 1:13 am, the tones sound. You and your partner are quick to respond to the scene, a local bar and grill. You arrive at the scene in less than 3 minutes in tandem with a police officer. Upon arrival, you find the remnants of what appears to have been a bar fight. The patient is a dazed male, approximately 26 years old, who obviously lost the fight. He is lying on his left side, drooling, and struggling to get to his feet. A quick assessment reveals a patent airway with a badly swollen and rapidly discoloring jaw, and a respiratory rate of 20 breaths/min. He agrees to let you check his vitals, which are found to be a heart rate of 146 beats/min. and a blood pressure of 106/58 mm Hg. He is placed under arrest on scene and transported by the police to the hospital and then the county jail. Nine months later, you receive a complaint naming you and your partner in a lawsuit alleging that you failed to obtain the patient's consent for treatment.

EMS providers are in a unique position compared to other members of the medical profession because they still routinely make house calls. Unlike every other medical provider, EMS providers are not only provided with the authority to practice medicine under the license and guidance of medical control, but they also possess—to a very limited extent—a degree of police-type powers that enable them to trespass on private property, violate certain traffic laws, and, under certain circumstances, transport a person against his or her will. EMS providers are commonly equipped with badges, lights, sirens, and uniforms, in addition to stethoscopes, blood pressure cuffs, and medical kits.

EMS providers who are just starting out in the field are likely to have an overwhelming feeling of excitement as well as uncertainty. Despite these feelings, the main concern of the provider is whether he or she is able to help the patient. Over the years, however, as EMS providers become seasoned, some become burnt out with their jobs. Their main focus gradually shifts. Rather than concerning themselves with what is best for the patient, other things take priority. For example, in an attempt to get back to the uneaten dinner waiting back at the station, a provider may rush through a call by just doing the bare minimum necessary to get that patient to the hospital. The line between the ancillary aspects of being an EMS provider and the obligations to the patient begin to blur.

Consent

Not only is ignoring a patient's full medical needs ethically wrong, it is illegal. The provider must remember, above all else, that the patient has the ultimate control and authority over the scene because the patient is always the EMS provider's primary concern. This premise is based on the statement from one of America's most famous and respected legal minds, Justice Benjamin Cardozo, in the 1914 case *Schoendorff v. Society of New York Hospital*. Cardozo stated that "every human being of adult years and sound mind has a right to determine what shall be done with his own body." This statement has become the foundation for the modern medical standard of informed consent. The "doctrine of informed consent" continues to be upheld and followed in all state and federal jurisdictions.

Most EMS providers think that the standard of informed consent is not applicable to their treatment because they provide "emergency" care. This is an incorrect presumption. In fact, in his ruling, Justice Cardozo addressed the emergency exception to informed consent, and held that consent must always be acquired, "except in cases of an emergency where the patient is unconscious, and where it is necessary to [administer medical treatment] before consent can be obtained." Therefore, according to established case law, it is mandatory for every medical provider to obtain informed consent before providing care to a conscious and coherent patient. By treating an individual without his or her consent, the medical provider may be committing **battery.**

The statutes and cases regarding informed consent laws have continued to evolve since Justice Cardozo's comments in 1914. Specifically, the cases have addressed the level of disclosure that a medical provider must provide when attempting to obtain informed consent. In doing so, two standards have emerged, with about half of the United States accepting one standard and the other half accepting the second. The first standard is the *prudent provider standard*. It states that the health care provider must disclose the same information regarding the care to be provided and the potential risks involved in receiving or not receiving treatment that any reasonable provider would disclose in a similar circumstance. The second standard is called the *reasonable patient standard*. This standard states that the health care provider must disclose a sufficient amount of information about the patient's care to allow a reasonable patient to make an informed decision.

Determining whether these standards have been met is legally considered to be a question of fact. At a trial, the attorneys present the evidence of expert testimony, but the jury holds the power to decide whether the information the provider disclosed to the patient before treating or obtaining a refusal was sufficient to meet either standard. The judge instructs the jury regarding which standard is applicable to the case. The

Legally Speaking

battery The unlawful touching of another individual without permission or excuse.

judge reaches his or her decision regarding which standard applies based on the case law of the state or federal jurisdiction where the court sits.

Disclosure of Information

What information should an EMS provider disclose? This question was answered in a famous case in 1970, *Canterbury v. Spence*. In this case, the court held that, ideally, a health care provider should disclose the *benefits, risks, and side effects of the treatment in addition to the alternatives to the treatment, and the consequences of no treatment*. After all of this information has been provided, the provider must then give the patient a choice as to whether or not he or she wants the treatment, as well as a choice as to what course of treatment the patient prefers. This court-imposed standard raises two questions for EMS providers. First, how can this practically be accomplished in the field setting? Second, what about those patients who are conscious but not competent?

Obtaining Consent

To address how an EMS provider can practically obtain consent while in the field, one can refer to how consent is obtained in the hospital setting. Usually, when a patient goes into the hospital for a surgical procedure, they undergo a consent process that includes discussion of the procedure. The physician does not disclose every minor detail related to the procedure, such as starting the intravenous (IV) line, taking vital signs, and administering a particular sedative as opposed to another. However, the physician should disclose any risks or potential adverse effects associated with a particular procedure or medication beforehand. If the patient is to undergo a surgical procedure, the physician should explain exactly what will be done during the surgery, the intended outcome, and the possible risks and adverse effects of the surgery. This approach can be applied to the EMS setting. After introductions are made, you should disclose to the patient that you would like to perform an evaluation, possibly start an IV to administer medications or replace lost fluids, and then transport him or her to the hospital. Then, ask if the patient has any questions. Listen to the patient. Do not merely proceed through this step as a formality. Ask for the patient's permission to perform the tasks you outlined previously. Finally, document the discussion and the patient's approval of your actions.

Following this consent procedure offers several benefits. First, it reduces your liability. Although anyone can attempt to sue for anything, the odds that the patient will be successful in a lawsuit are always reduced when proper procedures are followed and documented. Second, the consent procedure allows the patient to take an active role in his or her care. This has shown to benefit patient outcomes. Finally, following the consent procedure shows that you care about the patient and that you respect the patient and his or her condition. These qualities are a sign of professionalism and good customer service.

Legal Practices

Involving the family in the process of obtaining consent can be beneficial to an EMS provider on the scene. Family members often know what to say to convince the patient to accept treatment or be transported to the hospital. In addition, it may be more difficult for the patient to take legal action against the EMS provider for failure to obtain proper consent if the family was instrumental in the implementation of treatment. However, keep in mind that a family member cannot give consent on behalf of a patient who is refusing treatment unless such patient is a minor or incapacitated.

Implied Consent

In cases involving patients who are conscious but are not **competent** to make a decision regarding consent, the law holds that **implied consent** can be applied. Implied consent is a legally recognized doctrine that allows a provider to consider an unconscious or incoherent patient as having consented to treatment if a reasonable patient in the same circumstances would be presumed to give consent. The health care provider must then act in the best medical interests of the patient. Because your medical protocols have been designed in the best interest of the patient, strict adherence to your protocols is essential under implied consent.

There are three situations in which implied consent may be used. One such situation is when a patient is unconscious. Generally, there is not a problem with the immediate provision of care under this circumstance. However, the EMS provider should be aware of the possibility that a Do Not Resuscitate (DNR) order or a durable power of attorney may be in effect for the unconscious patient. The laws and procedures regarding the existence and enforcement of such orders vary state by state. (This topic is discussed in more detail later in this chapter.)

The second situation in which implied consent may be needed is if the patient is a minor. Generally, the law holds that minors are not legally competent to refuse or consent to medical care. In most jurisdictions, if a parent or guardian is not available to consent or refuse treatment for a minor child, it is presumed the parent would consent to care and care may be rendered under the doctrine of implied consent, even if the minor attempts to refuse. Although thorough documentation of the circumstances is a must, the provision of care should proceed in the same manner as directed by the medical protocols. Note, however, that some teenagers are considered legal adults under certain circumstances. **Emancipated minors** (for example, a teenager who is married) have been declared by the courts to have the legal capacity to make decisions as an adult. In these cases, the emancipated minor does have the ability to refuse treatment regardless of what a parent might say or what you might think is in the patient's best interests. Generally, such emancipated minors have some form of proof, such as a court-issued order, that verifies their emancipation.

The final situation in which care can be rendered without consent is when a patient is incompetent or lacks the capacity to grant consent. Whereas the legal doctrine of implied consent initially included people who were permanently mentally retarded, mute, or psychotic, the doctrine has been extended in most jurisdictions to include temporary incompetence secondary to intoxication from alcohol or drugs. In these circumstances providing care can be a difficult endeavor. Although the presence of police is recommended to ensure that you do not become injured, you do have the authority to treat a severely intoxicated patient or a psychotic patient without their consent. As always, consult your local protocol, as well as medical control, for specific treatment orders and guidelines regarding when you may deem patients mentally unfit to rely on their own consent. Also remember that proper documentation is imperative.

Legally Speaking

competent Mentally sound and free from undue burdens or external influences to make a decision; the mental capacity to make a decision.

implied consent The legal presumption that permission to render care in the patient's best interests is granted even though the patient is not competent to make an informed decision; occurs when a reasonable person in the same circumstances would be presumed to give consent.

emancipated minor A person younger than age 18 who is legally recognized by the court as having the authority to make his or her own decisions; to be treated legally as an adult.

Legal Practices

The legal status of an emancipated minor varies from state to state. You should always make sure you are familiar with the laws governing the particular jurisdiction in which you practice. Some states allow minors younger than age 18 to consent to medical treatment without being emancipated. Emancipation may also take place via the minor's status if he or she is younger than age 18 and married or serving in the armed forces.

Legally Speaking

Do Not Resuscitate (DNR) order
A legally binding order for health care providers to not provide life-saving measures during a cardiac or respiratory arrest; created at the request of the patient or the patient's legal designee.

Refusing Care

One of the most difficult parts of the EMS job is when a conscious and oriented patient refuses your care. For the average EMS provider who is trained under the theory that the actions he or she performs are always in the best interest of the patient, a refusal may not seem rational. Despite such personal feelings, an EMS provider must always respect a competent patient's refusal of medical treatment. The personal right of self-determination can be traced to the U.S. Constitution and is essential to the free and democratic society of which Americans are so proud. The Supreme Court has ruled that a patient has the right to refuse medical treatment, even if the patient's death is likely to be a direct result of the refusal. Failure to abide by a patient's request may lead to personal liability via assault and battery claims, false imprisonment charges, as well as civil rights claims.

If a patient refuses your care, you must first inform the patient of the consequences of the refusal, including the possibility of permanent injury or death. Second, you must confirm that the patient understands the consequences of the refusal. Have the patient explain back to you the potential problems that may arise if he or she does not allow you to proceed with treatment. Failure to understand the consequences could indicate that the patient is not competent. Finally, you should thoroughly document that you have informed the patient of the consequences and that the patient still refuses care. Be specific in your documentation; write down exactly what you told the patient and identify witnesses to your conversation.

It is best to have the patient sign the form or run report indicating that, despite being informed of all possible consequences, medical treatment has been refused. Most EMS agencies provide standardized, preprinted refusal forms. However, always keep in mind that a signature and checkmarks next to boxes on a preprinted form will not suffice to help you avoid liability without adequate descriptive documentation of the refusal. Along with thorough documentation, securing family members and police officers on the scene as witnesses to the refusal may support your defense should a lawsuit occur at a later time.

Do Not Resuscitate Orders

The same doctrine underlying a patient's right to refuse care provides the legal basis for the **Do Not Resuscitate (DNR) order.** Most states have DNR laws that govern the specifics of the process. DNR orders are generally used for patients with a terminal illness. These patients decide that if they go into cardiac or respiratory arrest, they do not want to receive any life-support measures. If a patient chooses to institute DNR orders, his or her primary health care provider follows the proper legal procedures required to issue a legally binding medical order that prohibits all providers from using advanced life support measures on that patient. The procedures involved in issuing a DNR are designed to ensure that such an order is truly based on the wishes of the patient or, in the case of an incapacitated patient, the patient's preestablished legally designated representative.

The technicalities of a DNR order vary from state to state. Whereas a DNR order in one state may restrict any advanced life support care, some states may provide for comfort care, such as pain-relieving medications and basic oxygen therapy. Some states may have a combination of provisions or may have different types of DNR orders based on what is permissible for that patient according to the patient's wishes. Further, each state has its own procedure for how to recognize a valid DNR order. Whereas some states rely on a written physician order, other states require the patient to wear a bracelet. Some states' DNR orders expire after a certain time frame and must be renewed in order to be considered valid. Most DNR orders are not valid outside of the state where they were issued. Make sure you check the specific statutes, regulations, and protocols governing your state and local region so that you are prepared for the time when you are presented with a DNR order. Most states require a copy of the signed and dated order to be present on scene in order for you to legally withhold potential lifesaving care. It is not adequate to simply rely on the word of family members or the patient's physician. If a patient's family member or physician claims that a DNR exists but can provide no legal documentation necessary to satisfy state standards, an EMS provider is obligated to treat the patient as if no such document exists.

Health Care Durable Power of Attorney and Living Wills

Similar to the DNR order, a **health care durable power of attorney** and a **living will** are documents that express a patient's wishes with respect to the provision of medical care should the patient not be able to express his or her wishes because of an incapacitating illness or injury. The documents differ from a DNR order in that a physician order to withhold medical care is not necessary, and the patient does not need to be diagnosed with a terminal illness to validate the documents. These documents are durable in the sense that they remain in effect when the patient becomes incompetent.

Generally, these documents are drafted or reviewed by an attorney under the direction of the patient. The documents legally allow a friend, relative, or guardian of the patient to make medical decisions on the patient's behalf. Each state has different laws regarding the production and enforcement of these documents. Based on many factors, including the availability of "do-it-yourself" legal documents on the internet and the general public becoming more educated in individual health care rights, the popularity of durable powers of attorney and living wills is increasing. Make sure you check the specific statutes, regulations, and protocols governing your state and local region so that you are prepared and know what you should do when presented with either of these documents.

Legally Speaking

health care durable power of attorney A legal document originated and signed by the patient that names a specific person to act on the patient's behalf to make medical decisions, including the withdrawal or withholding of care, should the patient be incapacitated and unable to make the required decisions.

living will A legal document originated and signed by the patient that provides specific instructions regarding the patient's wishes for the use of life-saving measures, including the withdrawal or withholding of care should the patient become incapacitated and unable to make or verbalize such decisions.

Confidentiality

Telling war stories is a definite part of EMS culture. Put a group of EMS providers in a room for more than five minutes and tall tales are bound to emerge. Additionally, the EMS setting, unlike the quiet, controlled setting of a physician's office or hospital room is one in which privacy is a rare commodity. Spectators, and sometimes even the press, can be found at most scenes.

Spectators and laypeople are drawn to the human drama and suffering that EMS providers face on a daily basis. Successful television shows, including *ER, Rescue 911, Paramedics,* and *Emergency!,* have been produced since the inception of EMS. Although the public's fascination with chasing ambulances, viewing crime scenes, and observing fires has, to some extent, fueled the demand for these shows and sparked more interest in EMS, these shows, through industry involvement and consultation, also serve as a medium through which public education grows. This can ultimately benefit the EMS field. The more the public knows about what EMS providers do and how they do it, the more likely they are to get support, cooperation, and even increased funding. However, the public's fascination with EMS calls can become detrimental if information presented infringes on patient confidentiality.

Ensuring the patient's confidentiality while maintaining positive public relations becomes a challenge for EMS providers. In tackling this issue, the provider must remember that the patient's confidentiality always comes first. If you are telling a story about a recent case, and you include information in your account that could identify a patient, you are potentially liable for several torts, including breach of confidentiality, negligent infliction of emotional distress, and, possibly, slander. As stated in Chapter 3, private medical information is legally protected information. Release of such information without proper consent may be considered a violation of the patient's civil rights.

Release of private medical information is governed by a myriad of federal and state laws, regulations, and case law. The federal Health Insurance Portability and Accountability Act (HIPAA), Public Law 104–191, 104th Cong., 21 August 1996, allows for the use of federal fines and criminal sanctions for wrongly disclosing a patient's private medical information. If you improperly disclose information or use a patient's private medical information in an improper manner, you could possibly face fines and prison as well as being sued civilly. HIPAA does allow for disclosure of protected health care information (PHI) in certain circumstances involving medical care, medical operations, or billing operations. Therefore, HIPAA restrictions should not interfere with your daily duties of treating and transporting patients, including your ability to transfer patient care documentation and other PHI-related information to and from receiving and sending facilities and other appropriate medical and billing personnel. HIPAA, however, does require each agency to have a designated privacy officer. The privacy officer is responsible for ensuring that all PHI—in written and electronic form—is kept secure and released only to authorized individuals or entities. Questions concerning HIPAA or the release of private information should be directed to your facility's privacy officer or counsel.

To protect yourself from liability, never disclose the name of a patient to anyone who is not directly related to the care of that patient. When you must have a conversation related to a patient, make sure you have privacy and that civilians cannot hear your conversation. The crowded elevator that takes you to the hospital cafeteria is not the place to discuss the patient that you just dropped off at the emergency department. In addition, try to avoid using patient names in radio transmissions. If you plan to use patient charts or other aids for educational purposes, remove all patient identifiers before distributing them. Such identifiers include patient photographs, initials, first and last names, residential addresses, and call or run numbers.

If you are concerned that the patient's identity might be revealed, obtain consent to the release of information from the patient before disclosure of the information. Make sure that the consent is written and obtained in a setting in which the patient is free from duress or pressure from outside influences, such as overbearing family members or staff making inappropriate threats regarding treatment or legal claims. It is recommended that you contact your facility's counsel to assist you with obtaining this consent.

A common situation in which patient confidentiality is breached is when a third-party layperson rides along on a run. In the 1986 court case, *Miller v. National Broadcasting Co.,* it was decided that the right of privacy trumps the freedom of the press. This case arose when an NBC television crew, doing a ride-along with a paramedic unit entered a home, filmed a code, and showed it on a television special without obtaining the consent of the family. The family was emotionally disturbed when they saw the report, so they sued the television network. The court held that when a television crew rides with an EMS unit, they are not allowed to enter a person's home to film unless they have consent to do so before entering the house. In order to film patient care in any setting, it is recommended that you obtain the patient's consent before filming the call.

Conclusion

Patients are the reason that EMS systems exist and EMS providers have jobs. Whereas EMS providers are eager to provide the best and highest level of medical care that their training, certification, and available technology allows, it is equally important for them to respect their patient's rights. There are three steps EMS providers can take to ensure they are respecting these rights:

1. Always obtain consent from all competent adults before providing care.
2. Always respect a patient's refusal of care, regardless of how contrary to your goals and job function it may seem.
3. Always ensure that the patient's identity and medical treatment remain confidential.

If you respect these patient rights, you will not only reduce your risk of liability, but you may also experience improved outcomes and increased satisfaction because your patients will appreciate your care and respect.

You Be the Judge

Discussion

Are you liable for failure to obtain consent? One could argue that the patient granted his consent to treatment when he allowed you to check his vital signs. Also, it could be argued that, once placed under arrest, the patient required medical clearance before heading off towards jail, which meant that the patient would be subject to another medical evaluation before being incarcerated, and evidence of deterioration of the patient's condition would be found and treated during that examination. Additionally, because the medical clearance would be performed with or without the patient's consent after he was arrested, the EMTs could argue that consent to their evaluation and treatment was implied. Other possible defenses include the fact that the patient was most likely intoxicated and unable to give informed consent, thus granting you implied consent.

In addition to possibly being liable for not obtaining consent, there is the legal issue of whether it was appropriate for you to leave the patient in the care and custody of the police after you performed your assessment instead of transporting the patient to the hospital in tandem with the police. Unless the police officers that took the patient to the hospital were of equal or greater certification than you, you may be liable for patient abandonment if you did not obtain an appropriate patient refusal of treatment.

The best way to defend yourself against a suit involving failure to obtain informed consent or an informed refusal is to take time at the scene to obtain that information. In addition, document all of your actions, including what you specifically told the patient, his specific responses to you, and the witnesses that were on scene. If the patient's level of intoxication prevents him from understanding and either consenting to or refusing treatment, you should follow the doctrine of implied consent and document all of your actions, the patient's responses, and the witnesses who were at the scene.

Bibliography

Canterbury v. Spence, 464 F.2d 772, 788–789 (D.C. Cir. 1970).

Miller v. National Broadcasting Co., 187 Cal. App. 3d 1463 (Cal. App. 2d Dist. 1986).

Schoendorff v. Society of New York Hospitals, 105 NE 92 (N.Y. 1914).

Medical Authority and Practice Acts

You Be the Judge

A volunteer EMS squad's chief is featured in a local newspaper article about what her organization does for the community. In the article, the chief is quoted as saying that, as an additional service, the squad's staff returns to the home of the patient a few days after a call to provide a follow-up health screening and check-up. The local prosecutor reads the article. Being a former EMT, the prosecutor believes that this is outside the scope of a certified EMT's practice. He files criminal charges against the chief and her colleagues for the practice of medicine without a license. What is the likely result of this action?

In order to practice medicine in the United States, one must meet the requirements of a particular state's **medical practice act.** If a person without official certification or formal permission renders health care services—regardless of how benign or basic the service may appear— that person is practicing medicine without a license and may be liable for criminal and civil penalties.

Medical Practice Acts

Based on the premise that most consumers of health care services are not specifically knowledgeable about the provision of health care, each state has exercised its **police powers** to make safe judgments about the competence of potential providers on behalf of its citizens. These decisions are conveyed to the public by the licensure and certification process. All facets of the health care industry are subject to this type of state regulation.

In theory, the license that a state provides is meant to indicate that an individual has a minimal competency of clinical skill in a given area. Health care providers are not the only professionals who are subject to state licensure laws. Lawyers, architects, engineers, cosmetologists, contractors, and others are also required to obtain a license in order to practice. Despite the standardization of licensure requirements within a provider's field, many commentators have suggested

Legally Speaking

medical practice act The state legislation that grants legal authority to a health care provider to practice in that state and dictates the provider's scope of practice and practice environment.

police powers The authority provided to states by the U.S. Constitution to adopt laws and conduct various acts to ensure public health and safety.

independent provider A healthcare provider who may provide medical care autonomously under the authority of his or her own license, as opposed to operating under the control of a licensed physician.

dependent provider A medical provider who provides certain care that falls under the same scope of practice as a physician, but requires medical oversight from a physician to render such care.

that licenses do more harm than good by complicating the provider's practice to the point that many qualified people stay out of the field or limit their practice.

Health care licensure attempts to create a balance between ensuring patients have access to competent patient care and restricting unqualified people from rendering health care services. Traditionally, due to the stronghold physicians have on the practice of medicine, allied health care providers have not been able to break into the market with much ease. The physician's power over who can practice medicine has been termed the "legalized monopoly." Even as recently as 1984, the American Medical Association, a professional association that provides an organized voice for physicians, was accused of preventing allied health care professions from expanding and developing their individual scopes of practice.

In many instances, medical practice acts have been all encompassing. For example, one state's statute defining medicine is considered to be so inclusive that providing aspirin to a friend for a headache or piercing someone's ear may be considered practicing medicine. A physician's medical license is so broad that it allows the physician to perform any medical act he or she desires, ranging from open heart surgery to a psychiatric consult, regardless of specialty or training.

Early on, allied health care providers (including EMS providers) faced the obstacle of gaining enough market power to convince legislators to alter the medical practice acts to allow their scopes of practice to be recognized.

One sign that indicated the allied health profession was gaining recognition was the classification of allied health providers as independent and dependent providers.

Independent Providers

Independent providers include chiropractors, podiatrists, and psychologists. In recognition of their value and autonomy, states have instituted independent boards of accreditation that oversee the licensure of these practitioners. These licenses permit independent providers to assume the practice of medical services without the direct oversight by a physician. Generally, the scope of these providers is outside that of what a traditional medical physician would provide.

Dependent Providers

Dependent providers, such as physician assistants (PAs), nurse practitioners (NPs), surgical assistants (SAs), certified nurse midwives, physical therapists, and EMS providers, render care that is within the same scope as physicians. Although in the past 20 years these dependent allied health care providers have gained a significant level of clinical autonomy, they still must receive medical oversight and supervision from physicians.

Dependent providers not only have to justify their right to practice, but they must also define their scope within the health care industry. The legal authority for EMS providers to render care is found within state statutes that are fairly comprehensive. These statutes vary from state to state.

Licensure Versus Certification

The scope of practice of the EMS provider is limited by many factors, including the major legislative issue of **certification** versus **licensure**. A license is distinctly different than a certification. For example, physicians are licensed to practice medicine, but may also seek a board certification for their specialty. The license, issued by the state, permits the practice of medicine, whereas a national, private, and independent board issues the certification attesting to additional competence.

The granting of a license, rather than certification, furnishes the provider with certain rights that are not always protected by certification, such as the guarantee of fair and equal treatment in disciplinary and investigative matters related to licensure (known as due process protection). In addition, licensure conveys a sense of autonomy that is essential in facilitating the practice of the given art as a clinician rather than a technician. Licensure also raises the level of a health care provider's accountability because all licensees are subject to the disciplinary actions of their respective licensing boards or commissions.

The differences between licensure and certification tend to be vague and are rarely clearly defined. *Black's Law Dictionary,* 6th edition (1990), defines license as "the permission by competent authority to do an act, which, without such permission, would be illegal, a trespass, a tort, or otherwise not allowable." *Black's Law Dictionary* defines certification as "the formal assertion of some fact." To put these definitions in the context of the EMS profession, certification is a process through which a person is granted the permission to use a title of an occupation or profession. The certification process does not indicate anything beyond minimal competence; it merely identifies that an individual possesses a certain level of credentials based on hours of training and examination. Because the certification process does not address training beyond minimal competency or specific skills within scopes of practice, certified EMS providers usually require medical oversight by a licensed professional.

Licensure connotes a level of autonomy within a given industry. Moreover, the right to practice that is inherent with the license is usually deemed by the courts to be a property right that is subject to due process as afforded by the Constitution. (See Chapter 10 for more information about due process.)

The majority of the states use certification for EMS providers, but some states have started licensing providers. This has enabled EMS providers to expand their autonomy and scope of practice, which may also expand their liability.

Scope of Practice

As dependent providers, EMS professionals are taught that their role is to perform emergency medical care—not to practice medicine. EMS providers should serve as the physician's eyes and ears in the field. Paramedic textbooks continue to instruct students that, despite the vast range of technical skills that they are authorized to perform, the paramedic

Legally Speaking

certification Evidence of level of training; the formal assertion of some fact.

licensure The right to practice; the permission by competent authority to perform an act, which, without such permission, would be illegal, a trespass, a tort, or otherwise not allowable.

Legally Speaking

scope of practice The level and type of care that a provider may legally render based on state statute and local protocols.

still has no independent authority to provide any medical care or make any diagnosis regarding a patient's condition. Any care rendered by a certified paramedic is legally considered to be an extension of the licensed physician under whom the paramedic works.

Some physicians continue to try to expand EMS providers' **scope of practice** under their license by seeking to allow the EMS providers to practice in an emergency department, private practice, or home health care setting. The Court of Appeals of Arizona recently addressed this practice in *Hospital Corporation of Northwest, Inc. v. Arizona Department of Health Services.* In this case, Northwest Hospital Corporation in Arizona (*Northwest*) used paramedics in its emergency department to facilitate patient care. The paramedics were dispensing drugs, such as Tylenol™, Mylanta™, and ibuprofen. These drugs were not approved by the Arizona Department of Health Services (DHS) for administration by paramedics.

Northwest contended that, first, paramedics should be able to enjoy an expanded scope of practice when under physician supervision. Second, Northwest argued that the DHS regulations were solely applicable to the field setting. The DHS disagreed, arguing that if state statute grants the DHS the authority to regulate the education, training, certification, and discipline of paramedics, it is also the only agency that has the authority to delineate the scope of practice for EMS providers. Further, the health department contended that such delineation is applicable to any role in which a paramedic practices. The Court of Appeals held that the DHS has the statutory authority to perform all such actions, and that "a paramedic who works . . . where physicians are present does not enjoy an enlarged scope of practice simply because the hospital wishes it so." This holding has had a significant impact on the utilization of certified providers under medical supervision in a clinical environment as a way to reduce costs.

A similar ruling in Virginia determined that a paramedic's role is not considered to change depending on the setting where he or she practices. In the case *Mercy Tidewater Ambulance Service v. Carpenter,* it was stated that "although the jobs were performed in different settings (ie, an ambulance versus an emergency room), the employments were (held to be of) the same general class."

The case of *Schultz v. Rural/Metro Corp.* further complicated the issue of the EMS provider's role as an agent of the medical control physician's license. In this case, the Texas Court of Appeals held that a medical transport company was not an agent of its medical director. Additionally, the court went so far as to say that the EMS service was not even a "health care provider." (It should be noted that this case revolved around the definition of a healthcare provider.) Although such a distinction has not affected how EMS providers deliver patient care in Texas, it may have had some consequences regarding the level of protection that EMS providers are afforded by medical immunity statutes.

As the above cases illustrate, states vary in what is included in your scope of practice. If it seems that your medical director is being restrictive, keep in mind that your state's laws may be what is prohibiting you from enjoying an expanded scope of practice.

Legal Practices

The scope of practice varies not only state by state, but also varies by county or region within the state, depending on your medical directors and their interpretation of your state's regulations. Be proactive in becoming aware of your scope of practice. Encourage a meeting with your medical director to understand the restrictions of your certification or license in each particular setting.

Medical Control

The role of medical control is to provide a direct connection between EMS providers and the licensed physician under whom they practice. It is a vital element of an EMS system because an EMS provider is not permitted to practice without such medical direction. Attempts to provide medical services without medical control may be construed as practice of medicine without a license.

Medical control is exercised by a medical director who has the ultimate authority over the scope of an EMS provider's care. The medical director oversees education and quality assurance and should personally know the providers who work under his or her supervision.

There are two forms of medical control: **online medical control** and **off-line medical control.** Online medical control occurs when an EMS provider is in direct contact with the authorized physician, either via telephone or radio communications or in person, and patient specific information is being discussed. Off-line medical control occurs when an authorized physician provides such services as continuing medical education, medical guidance, and practice guidelines. For example, the medical control physician provides the EMS agency with the medical protocols—guidelines and practice pathways that dictate how and to what extent the EMS providers are able to provide medical care. Traditionally, it has been thought that the guidelines or protocols simply define the skills the providers can render under the auspice of the physician's medical license. However, this form of off-line medical control is also used when direct, online control is unavailable or impractical under the circumstances.

Although the term supervision may connote a direct and close working relationship between a physician and the EMS provider, supervision has generally been interpreted to mean the mere communication between the two. Immediate supervision, in which a physician is standing over the provider and directing the provider's actions, is not cost efficient. In addition, immediate supervision does not correlate with the health care industry's intended goals of using EMS providers. What is the minimal level of supervision required? In the federal case *MacDonald v. United States,* a court held that a military medical facility that required physicians to check approximately 10% of the cases treated by a physician's assistant did not provide enough supervision. The court further stated that this level of supervision was "inadequate" and the facility illegally permitted physician's assistants to practice in an expanded scope of care.

> **Legally Speaking**
>
> **online medical control** Patient-specific medical guidance, direction, or authorization that occurs through direct, immediate contact between the physician and the EMS provider.
>
> **off-line medical control** Medical guidance, direction, or authorization provided by a physician before patient care is rendered; can be relied on in cases where online medical control is not available.

Dealing With Other Physicians on Scene

In many cases, a physician with whom you are not familiar will appear on scene as a Good Samaritan and then start giving you orders. It is extremely important that you follow your department's policies or procedures for handling such a situation. Although the physician does have a medical license (a fact that should be validated by asking the person to show you his or her wallet-sized license card), you should state that you are not authorized to work under his or her license. Remind the physician that should he or she treat the patient, he or she will legally be considered to assume care of the patient. This will require the physician to travel with the patient in the ambulance to the hospital in order to avoid illegally abandoning the patient. Assisting the physician with any actions if he or she refuses to assume full responsibility for the patient's care may put you, as well as the physician, in legal jeopardy. Therefore, you should not assist such physicians in delivering medical treatment or follow any orders given unless he or she assumes full patient care. Furthermore, even if the physician does assume patient care, you must never provide or assist in providing care that is outside of your scope of practice or that you deem to be contrary to the patient's best medical interest.

As with all occurrences of unusual circumstances, a situation such as this should be thoroughly documented. It is also recommended that you establish online medical control as soon as possible. If medical control advises you to do so, you may assist the on-scene physician with actions within your scope of practice and protocols while remaining under the authority of your medical control physician.

Conclusion

The practice of medicine is a privilege. You should respect and appreciate the authority you have been given by the state and your local medical director to provide medical care. Although you do not have the proper medical licensure or authority to practice without medical control, this does not indicate that the care that you do provide is not valuable and cannot make a difference. The scope of practice of the EMS provider is addressed in state statutes as well as medical protocols. If you adhere to medical control at all times, you will be able to render care with a minimal amount of liability.

You Be the Judge

Discussion

Whether the criminal charges of practicing medicine without a license can be successfully prosecuted depends on three factors.

First, what is actually involved in "a follow-up health screening and check-up?" Does it involve invasive procedures or just an assessment of vital signs? How is the information obtained during this check-up used? Are the squad members engaged in activity that could be deemed "diagnosing" or are they merely reporting the vital signs obtained to the patient for his or her own reference?

Second, what is the level of certification of the squad members conducting this "health screening and check-up?" Are the individuals conducting these exams certified as basic EMTs, paramedics, or something else?

And finally, what are the specific terms of the medical practice act of the state involved? If the actual procedures being done are within the provider's scope of EMS practice guidelines and protocols for his or her certification level and do not meet the definition of "diagnosing" or any other activity that is prohibited for unlicensed physicians by the state's medical practice act, the prosecutor will not be able to go forward with his case. If the activity that comprises the "health screening and check-up" are beyond the provider's regular scope of practice protocols or violate specific provisions of the state's medical practice act, the prosecutor would most likely be successful in his case.

Bibliography

Hospital Corporation of Northwest, Inc. v. Arizona Department of Health Services, 295 Ariz. Adv. Rep 17, 988 P.2d 168 (1999).

MacDonald v. United States, 853 F. Supp. 1430, 1438 (M.D. Ga. 1994).

Mercy Tidewater Ambulance Service v. Carpenter, 29 Va. App. 218, 511 S.E.2d 418 (1999).

Schultz v. Rural/Metro Corp., 956 S.W.2d 757 Tex. App., 14th Dist. (1997).

Chapter 6

Good Samaritan Laws and Immunities

You Be the Judge

Bill, a certified paramedic, keeps a full advanced life support jump kit in his private vehicle. Bill would like to have a top-of-the line cardiac monitor/defibrillator, but it would be too expensive. However, Bill has purchased an automatic external defibrillator (AED), which he keeps with his equipment. He often stops at accident scenes to offer help. One day, he encounters a teenage pedestrian who was struck by a car. Being the first on scene, Bill starts care. He figures that because he is a paramedic and he has all of the necessary equipment, he will call 9-1-1 after he stabilizes the patient. Bill assesses correctly that the patient has a pneumothorax that is quickly turning into a tension pneumothorax. Bill takes out a chest tube kit that he "procured" from the local emergency department and begins to insert a chest tube. During the procedure, however, Bill cuts an artery and the pedestrian dies from hypovolemic shock. The patient's parents sue. Bill claims that he is a Good Samaritan. What is the likely result of the suit?

Up until the turn of the twentieth century, patients generally did not hold health care providers accountable for undesired outcomes associated with the delivery of medical services. This is not true today. Accountability of health care providers is an increasingly important topic. Fueled by more aggressive tort claims and increased fiscal pressures, the health care provider no longer enjoys the complete autonomy experienced at the turn of the twentieth century.

In 1982, the case *Andrews v. United States* established the current legal precedent that holds medical providers liable for acts that do not meet the standards of a reasonable health care provider at the same level of training when they are faced with similar circumstances. This important concept suggests that EMS providers are liable for care rendered within the scope of the EMS provider's practice; not for the standard of care set by what another provider, such as an emergency department nurse or physician assistant (PA), may provide. This precedent was later applied in the case *Paris v. Kreitz,* which held that a PA was not liable for the same standard of practice as a medical doctor.

However, as EMS embarks upon a new era in health care delivery, the current standards may change. Actions EMS providers were previously immune from are now, in some instances, actions for which they may be held accountable. This chapter is designed to provide insight on how changes in accountability standards impact the EMS profession.

History of Good Samaritan Laws

Prehospital emergency medicine is one of the few professions in which some form of immunity from negligent acts is automatically provided to its members. The specifics of such blanket immunity vary from state to state, but the development of immunity legislation was triggered by the almost universally accepted Good Samaritan laws. Good Samaritan laws are designed to eliminate the common-law right of a victim of an emergency to pursue legal action for negligent acts performed by a physician who voluntarily and without compensation renders aid. Whereas these laws were initially designed to encourage physicians to stop and provide medical assistance in the event of an emergency, the support for this policy has grown to encompass first aid rendered by nonmedically trained rescuers. Between 1960 and 1982, all fifty states and the District of Columbia enacted a form of this law. (For a list of the Good Samaritan laws, see Table 6.1.) Legislators intended for the Good Samaritan laws to encourage people to provide assistance at the scene of an emergency without the fear of potential liability.

Table 6.1
Listing of State Good Samaritan Laws
Ala. Code § 6-5-332 (Supp. 1981)
Alaska Stat. § 09.65.090 (Supp. 1980)
Ariz. Rev. Stat. Ann. § 32-1471 (West Supp. 1981)
Ark. Stat. Ann. § 72-624 (Supp. 1979)
Cal. Bus. & Prof. Code §§ 2395-2398 (West Supp. 1981)
Colo. Rev. Stat. § 13-21- 108 (Supp. 1976)
Conn. Gen. Stat. § 52-557b (1980)
D.C. Code Ann. § 2-142 (Supp. V 1978)
Del. Code Ann. Tit. 16, § 6801-6802 (Supp. 1980)
Fla. Stat. Ann. § 768.13 (West Supp. 1982)
Ga. Code § 84-930 (1981)
Hawaii Rev. Stat. § 663-1.5 (Supp. 1979)
Idaho Code § 5-330 (1979)
Ill. Ann. Stat. Ch. 111, § 4404 (Smith-Hurd 1981)
Ind. Code Ann. § 34-4-12-1 (Burns 1973)
Iowa Code Ann. § 613.17 (West Supp. 1981)
Kan. Stat. Ann. § 65-2891 (1980)
Ky. Rev. Stat. § 411.148 (Supp. 1980)
La. Rev. Stat. Ann. §§ 37:1731-1732 (West 1980)
Me. Rev. Stat. Ann. Tit. 14, § 164 (1980)
Md. Ann. Code Art. 43, § 132 (Supp. 1981)
Mass. Ann. Laws Ch. 112, § 12b (Michie/Law Co-Op. 1975)
Mich. Comp. Laws Ann. § 691.1501 (Supp. 1981)

(continued)

Table 6.1 (continued)

Minn. Stat. Ann. § 604.05 (West Supp. 1981)
Miss. Code Ann. § 73-25-37 (Supp. 1981)
Mo. Ann. Stat. § 190.195 (Vernon Supp. 1981)
Mont. Code Ann. § 17-410 (1967)
Neb. Rev. Stat. § 25-1152 (1979)
Nev. Rev. Stat. § 41.500 (1980)
N.M. Rev. Stat. Ann. § 508.12 (Supp. 1979)
N.J. Stat. Ann. § 2a:62a-1 (West Supp. 1980)
N.M. Stat. Ann. § 24-10-3 To -4 (1976)
N.Y. Educ. Law § 6527(2) (Mckinney Supp. 1981)
N.C. Gen. Stat. § 20-166(D) (1978)
N.D. Cent. Code §§ 43-17-37 To -38 (1978)
Ohio Rev. Code Ann. § 2305.23 (Page 1981)
Okla. Stat. Ann. Tit. 76, § 5 (West. Supp. 1981)
Or. Rev. Stat. § 30.800 (1979)
42 Pa. Cons. Stat. Ann. §§ 8331-2 (Purdon 1981)
R.I. Gen. Laws § 5-37-14 (1976)
S.C. Code Ann. § 15-1-310 (Law. Co-Op. 1976)
S.D. Codified Laws Ann. § 20-9-3 (1979)
Tenn. Code Ann. § 63-622 (Supp. 1981)
Tex. Stat. Ann. Art. La (Vernon Supp. 1981)
Utah Code Ann. § 58-12-23 (Supp. 1981)
Vt. Stat. Ann. Tit. 12, § 519(B) (1973)
Va. Code § 8.01-225 (Supp. 1981)
Wash. Rev. Code Ann. § 4.24.300 (Supp. 1981)
W. Va. Code § 55-7-15 (1981)
Wis. Stat. Ann. § 448.06(7) (West Supp. 1981)
Wyo. Stat. § 33-26-143 (1977)

Source: Collected from the actual legislative materials for each jurisdiction by the author.
KEY: § = section; Ann. = Annotated; Rev. = Revised; Stat. = Statutes; Supp. = Supplement

The expansion of Good Samaritan laws eventually grew to specifically incorporate career emergency medical professionals. Although the degree of protection differs between the states, the underlying effect is that EMS providers in most jurisdictions throughout the United States enjoy some form of immunity from liability for negligent actions. Table 6.2 summarizes the current Good Samaritan legislation for every state.

Thirteen states do not provide any type of civil immunity for EMS providers. Nineteen states have broad, sweeping legislation that gives providers, instructors, and supervisors immunity for any negligent act or omission. One state, Alaska, only provides this type of immunity for the providers. Six states provide complete immunity for all involved (providers, instructors, and supervisors) in emergency situations only. Four states provide immunity only when off-duty personnel provide the care without cost. Delaware is the one state that only provides immunity for paramedics. The remaining states provide various immunity provisions, such as for automatic external defibrillator use (Montana), volunteer providers (Vermont), and instructors (Connecticut, Delaware, and Maine).

Table 6.2

Good Samaritan Laws Liability Limits

State	Limits on Liability
AL	4
AK	2
AZ	6
AR	N
CA	1
CO	N
CT	6
DE	5, 6
DC	1
FL	1
GA	4
HI	N
ID	1
IL	1
IN	1
IA	4
KS	3
KY	4
LA	1
ME	6
MD	N
MA	1
MI	1
MN	1
MO	3
MS	N
MT	8
NE	1
NV	N
NH	3
NM	N
NJ	1
NY	9
NC	N
ND	1
OH	1
OK	N
OR	3
PA	N
RI	1
SC	N
SD	3
TN	1
TX	1
UT	1
VT	7
VA	3
WA	N
WV	1
WI	N
WY	4

KEY: 1 = All providers, instructors, and supervisors are immune from negligent acts or omissions; 2 = All providers are immune from negligent acts or omissions; 3 = All providers, instructors, and supervisors are immune from negligent acts or omissions in an emergency situation; 4 = Providers who render free care are immune from negligent acts or omissions in an emergency situation; 5 = Paramedics are immune from negligent acts; 6 = Instructors are immune; 7 = Volunteer personnel are immune from negligent acts; 8 = Immunity from using an AED; 9 = Immunity for DNR violation; N = Not mentioned

Illinois has ruled that if an EMS provider passes the closest hospital or medical facility in order to take a patient to an alternative location, it is an act that is willful or wanton. Therefore, if a provider does not take the patient to the closest hospital, he or she may be held liable for gross negligent behavior, and thus will not be immune. (See Chapter 7 for more information on negligent behavior.)

In the District of Columbia, immunity from civil actions is the only provision that relates to EMS personnel. The law provides immunity for providers within the scope and duty of their practice.

Will a Court Really Uphold Immunity for an EMS Provider?

Most Good Samaritan statutes say that when a patient files a negligence lawsuit against an EMS provider, the court should simply dismiss the case without a trial unless gross negligence or intentional civil wrongs are alleged.

Similar to most states, New Jersey includes a provision in its laws that excludes liability for civil damages that occur after an EMS provider's actions, as long as such actions are in "good faith and in accordance" with the provisions in the licensing statute. *Frields v. St. Joseph's Hospital and Medical Center* demonstrates the judiciary's willingness to uphold the civil immunity of an EMS provider. In this case, the EMS providers failed to adequately assess the patient because of his combative nature. The patient died from a head injury, a condition for which combativeness or altered level of consciousness are signs. A motion judge (a judge of a lower court, such as a district court) ruled that the mobile intensive care unit personnel were immune from liability under the New Jersey statute. The Superior Court of New Jersey affirmed this decision.

However, not all jurisdictions are as generous as New Jersey in their interpretation as to what is considered "acting in good faith." For example, in *Zinger v. The City of Lynn,* decided in 1995, the United States First District Court refused to apply the Massachusetts EMS negligence immunity statute to automatically dismiss a negligence case against two EMTs whose patient died from cardiac arrest after being restrained face down on a stretcher. Instead, the court held that EMTs who placed the restrained psychiatric patient face down on the stretcher may not have necessarily acted in "good faith." Therefore, the question of negligence would have to be resolved at trial. Another blow to the Massachusetts EMS negligence immunity statute occurred with the case *Musto v. Cataldo.* The Massachusetts Suffolk Superior Court of Suffolk County held that the Massachusetts EMS negligence immunity statute does not apply to EMTs during routine hospital-to-hospital transports; it only applies to emergency situations.

Effects of Immunity

Studies documenting the effectiveness of the Good Samaritan laws are scarce, but some authorities argue that this immunity can be harmful to the patient. In a recent study that surveyed members of the American

Law and Economics Association, 67% of respondents thought that it is inefficient to hold Good Samaritans immune for negligent rescue.

In many large cities with high call volumes, some EMS providers have been known to rely on their immunity status to take short cuts without fear of the consequences their negligent acts may cause. For example, patients with suspected heart attacks or traumatic injuries might be walked to the ambulance rather than carried in an effort to save time. Such a short cut can have severe implications. In the case of a suspected heart attack patient, the additional strain that can occur with walking down stairs can increase the size and severity of the damage to the heart muscle. If a victim of traumatic injury has a spinal cord injury that was not identified by the EMS provider, moving the patient improperly could lead to paralysis.

The Future of Immunity

In the early years of EMS, the majority of the providers volunteered their time and skills. Volunteers were used because EMS systems did not have the adequate resources to compensate personnel. Immunity for these providers encouraged volunteerism, which gave communities the opportunity to be able to afford to provide some type of EMS. In *Jennings v. Southwood* and *Boroditsch v. Community Emergency Medical Service, Inc.,* the court held that immunity is necessary to encourage people to function as EMS providers. However, the growth and popularity of EMS has led to the emergence of systems into every community across the country, and additional resources are available to compensate providers. Today, the majority of EMS is performed by compensated, career providers, not volunteers with minimal resources. Offering immunity as an incentive to attract these quality providers may not be as valid as it once was. Some argue that shifting from immunity to accountability for the care rendered to a patient is understandable and practical.

There is some evidence that the current levels of immunity are already diminishing. The number of suits against EMS providers is projected to increase with the expansion of the scopes of practice of many EMTs. Therefore, accountability for EMS providers' acts may be justified by these broader scopes of practice, the transformation of EMS agencies from volunteer services to career agencies, and the more stringent educational standards in place for today's EMS provider.

Efforts to increase accountability and reduce immunity may have some positive effects on the EMS field. Through increased accountability, the industry may be required to increase educational requirements, demonstrate positive outcomes, and justify providers' scopes of practice. Currently, EMS providers, depending on jurisdictional regulations, provide some of the most invasive procedures of all allied health providers with the least comprehensive educational requirements. Increasing accountability, education, and training standards similar to other health care providers may be the catalyst for various system changes, including outcome-related research, licensure, and professional recognition. All of these reforms could help transform the image of the EMS provider from that of a technician and ambulance driver to that of a respected clinician of emergency medicine.

Protecting Immunity and Reducing Liability

For now, immunity is a valuable resource for EMS providers and should be respected as such. However, preemptive action should be taken now, such as modifying risk-management plans and obtaining advisory opinions from attorneys general, to enact a system that will be able to handle the potential increasing risk of liability. What can you do to reduce your potential liability? Remember the legal ABCs of EMS: **A**lways document; **B**e kind; and **C**ontact medical control. (See Chapter 3 for more information about the legal ABCs.)

Legal Practices

1. You should know to what extent your state provides immunity because the levels of immunity vary from state to state. Check not only your state's statutes, but also the administrative code.

2. If you do provide care off duty, as a private citizen or "Good Samaritan," you should still document the entire call just as if you were providing care on duty. Mail a copy of the documentation to your medical director. Doing so will help legitimize your documentation and reduce your exposure to liability.

3. When providing care as a Good Samaritan, do not exceed first responder or basic life support services, regardless of your level of training or intent. Providing care beyond these levels may negate the immunity to which you may be entitled.

Conclusion

Historically, EMS providers have been immune from liability for matters of simple negligence. This was initially meant to encourage EMS providers to serve their communities, but some legal analysts now argue that immunity has become a crutch for providers and may even have negative effects on patient care. As the field of EMS grows and evolves, it is projected that the doctrine of immunity will slowly decline. Therefore, in order to decrease liability, providers should follow their local protocols and agency policies, act within their scope of practice and medical control, and treat all patients with respect and professionalism.

You Be the Judge

Discussion

Whether Bill is considered a Good Samaritan under these circumstances depends on the statute of the jurisdiction where the event occurred. First and foremost, the determining factor would be the language of the existing Good Samaritan statute for that state, assuming there is such a statute.

Assuming such law exists in the jurisdiction, the next question would be whether Bill "acted in good faith." Stopping to help an injured person at the scene of an accident while off duty certainly appears to be "acting in good faith." However, if the procedure Bill performed is not within his scope of practice and he did not have online or off-line medical control to perform such a procedure, most courts would find that the actions were not in "good faith," and Bill would not be afforded the immunity. The fact that the chest tube was not a standard issue piece of equipment, but was "procured" from a hospital also hurts Bill's case and increases his liability.

Bibliography

Andrews v. United States, 548 F.Supp. 603, 610 (D.S.C. 1982).

Boroditsch v. Community Emergency Medical Service, Inc., 521 N.W.2d 230 (1994).

Frields v. St. Joseph's Hospital and Medical Center, 305 N.J. Super. 244, 702 A.2d 353 (1997).

Jennings v. Southwood, 446 Mich 125, 521 N.W.2d 230 (1994).

Musto v. Cataldo, Mass. Super. Lexis 456 (1995).

Paris v. Kreitz, 331 S.E.2d 234, 247 (N.C. App. 1985).

Zinger v. The City of Lynn, 875 F.Supp. 53, (1995).

Chapter 7

Negligence

You Be the Judge

Jennifer, a state-certified EMT-Basic, is providing care to an unresponsive, unconscious patient who has an unstable airway. She and her EMT partner are the first on the scene. Paramedics are en route. In her state, the new Department of Transportation (DOT) National Curriculum for EMT-Basics has been adopted, which means Jennifer is allowed to intubate. She successfully intubates the patient. After intubation, she and her partner verify tube placement and document their actions. The patient is then lifted onto a stretcher and put in the back of the ambulance. Paramedics still have not arrived on scene. Jennifer and her partner begin to drive to the hospital and agree to meet the paramedics halfway. Fifteen minutes elapse between the intubation and the time that the paramedics catch up with Jennifer and her patient en route to the hospital. At that time, the patient is cyanotic and pulseless. Despite their best efforts, the patient dies. When the chart is reviewed, there is nothing mentioned in the documentation about assessment of the airway after each time they moved the patient or while en route to the hospital. Is Jennifer negligent? To what extent is she liable?

EMS varies from place to place and system to system. Some departments are large career systems with multimillion dollar budgets. Other departments rely on the generosity of the local citizens to volunteer their time so that the ambulance can be staffed during peak hours. Some systems have brand new state-of-the-art vehicles and equipment, whereas others rely on duct tape to keep the equipment together so it can last another budget cycle.

Regardless of what system you work in, as a medical provider you have certain responsibilities and obligations. Overall, you are required to provide medical care to the standard that a reasonable provider who is certified at the same level would provide under a similar set of circumstances. In the EMS world, it is easy to define what this standard is because of the use of medical protocols. It is your duty to provide care that is consistent with such medical protocols.

Failure to act according to your duty can create liability. Liability can be criminal, wherein the state seeks retribution on behalf of society for a wrong that you caused, or civil, wherein the injured party seeks retribution and restitution. Civil harms are referred to as **torts,** and a person who commits a tort is known as a **tortfeasor.** Nonintentional harms are known as negligent torts, which are discussed in this chapter. If you choose to purposely disobey or deviate from the standard, then the liability is in the form of an intentional tort. Intentional torts are covered in Chapter 8.

Elements of a Negligent Tort

A tort that occurs without intent to do harm is a negligent tort. In order to prove that a defendant has committed a negligent act, the plaintiff (the injured party) has the burden to prove four elements:

1. The defendant had a duty to the plaintiff;
2. The defendant breached such duty;
3. Actual harm occurred to the plaintiff;
4. The injury was substantially caused by the breach of such duty.

In order for someone to be found negligent, all four elements must be present, and it must be proven that it is more likely than not that they occurred.

Of these four elements, duty is the easiest for the plaintiff to prove. Certain factors infer a duty on your part. These may include being on duty, wearing a uniform, having a current license or certification, or being dispatched to a call and acknowledging the dispatch. The standard of care and the scope of your duty as a health care provider are defined by the medical protocols and standard operating procedures that are issued to you.

Once duty is demonstrated, the plaintiff has to prove that a breach of the duty occurred. To do this, the plaintiff uses various forms of evidence, including, but not limited to, the testimony of witnesses, other EMS providers who were at the scene, and hospital personnel; the medical record from the incident; tape recordings of radio communications; computer-aided dispatch records; and a copy of your facility's medical protocols and standard operating procedures. These pieces of evidence may be used to demonstrate that you deviated from your responsibility as an EMS provider.

For example, you and your partner have just finished a call. You indicate that you are available by hitting the proper command on your computer-aided dispatch (CAD) console unit inside your vehicle. As you hit the button, you and your partner pull into a local sandwich shop to grab dinner. Immediately after you order, you are dispatched to a call for a patient complaining of chest pain. Rather than canceling your order, you wait until your food is ready. You place the sandwiches between the two front seats (which is against Occupational Safety and Health Administration [OSHA] regulations, unless the cab is completely separate from the patient compartment) and finally respond eight minutes after you were initially dispatched. You indicate your response by hitting the appropriate

Legally Speaking

tort A private or civil wrong or injury resulting from a breach of a legal duty that exists by virtue of society's expectations regarding interpersonal conduct rather than by contract or other private relationship.

tortfeasor A person who commits a tort.

Legally Speaking

burden of proof The duty of a party to substantiate an allegation to avoid the dismissal of that issue, or to convince the trier of facts regarding the truth of a claim in order to prevail in a civil or criminal suit.

preponderance of the evidence A degree of evidence that suggests that a person is more likely to be liable for harm than not; proof which leads the trier of fact to find that the existence of the fact in issue is more probable than not.

key on the CAD unit. Upon arrival, the patient is in cardiac arrest. Your attempts to resuscitate fail.

Eighteen months later, you are served with a lawsuit claiming that you are liable for the patient's death. During discovery, the CAD reports indicating that there was an eight-minute delay between dispatch and response are entered into evidence, along with the testimony of the worker from the sandwich shop. The plaintiff's case states that you had a duty to respond immediately upon being given the information of the call. You were available, and you breached your duty by waiting to get your food.

The plaintiff next has to prove an injury. In the above example, is the patient's death the injury? Not necessarily. In this case, the decreased chance of survival needs to be examined in order to determine the legal existence of an actual injury. According to the American Heart Association's advanced cardiac life support guidelines, immediate defibrillation is the best treatment for resuscitation of cardiac arrest. The plaintiff may attempt to argue that during the eight minutes that you delayed your response, the patient's chance for survival was most likely greatly decreased. However, not all cardiac arrest patients are candidates for defibrillation, so expert witnesses will have to study the available information regarding the electrical activity in the deceased heart at time of death and provide an expert opinion as to whether the delayed response would have made a difference in the patient's survival.

In some circumstances, however, the death is considered the injury. If you administered the wrong medication because you failed to check it properly before administration, and the patient's death was caused by an adverse reaction to the medication, the injury is considered the death. However, injuries do not need to be so dramatic to elicit a lawsuit. If you dropped a patient, you may be liable for the resulting injury, such as a fractured pelvis or even just bruising and delayed recovery.

Finally, the plaintiff must show that the injury sustained was directly related to your breach of duty. Thus, if you dropped the patient, you would be liable for the subsequent broken pelvis, but not the fractured ankle that was the patient's chief complaint for which you were treating. In the case of the cardiac arrest patient, the decreased chance of survival was directly related to the delay that you caused by waiting for the sandwiches, and thus, the injury would be directly related to your breach of duty.

Burden of Proof

Because a negligence tort is a civil matter that is heard in a civil court of law, the plaintiff's **burden of proof** is to prove the presence of the four negligence elements by a **preponderance of the evidence.** This means that the plaintiff tries to prove that it was more likely than not that the four elements of neglect occurred. Although the legal world does not like to place numbers to legal theory, this burden of proof has been described as a 51% likelihood that the four elements happened. If the plaintiff proves that there was a 51% likelihood that in a specific situation you had a duty, you breached that duty, an injury occurred, and that the injury was caused by your breach of duty, the burden shifts to you to provide a defense.

Defenses

A defense is a justification as to why the act that caused the harm may not create liability for the defendant. The defense is presented after the plaintiff proves the four elements of negligence. One type of defense used is called an affirmative defense. This type uses an established theory that is based on case law as a defense. If an applicable affirmative defense is provided, the plaintiff's case collapses.

The most common affirmative defense used for those in the EMS field is **immunity.** There are two types of immunity. The first arises from the state's Good Samaritan laws. In this sort of immunity, the EMS provider is expressly protected from the lawsuit by the statutory provision of the region in which the civil action occurred.

The second type of immunity is **sovereign immunity.** The concept of sovereign immunity originated in the old English common law when it was determined that an individual could not sue the king. In the American legal system, the theory of sovereign immunity states that the government is immune from most civil liability. Many states continue to rely on this theory in order to prevent the state's public treasury from being reduced by payments to private individuals who might prevail in lawsuits against the state. Therefore, in such states, EMS systems that are contracted by the government are immune from liability. In some states, however, the legal premise of sovereign immunity has been abandoned, thus leaving the EMS provider with immunity only as designated by the state EMS immunity provision, if applicable.

An additional type of defense is called **contributory negligence.** This defense is based on the assumption that the injured patient's actions led to or significantly contributed to the breach of duty that caused the injury. In the case of a patient who is dropped, if the patient was conscious, alert, oriented, and moving around excessively despite your requests to remain still, the EMS provider could argue that the patient's actions contributed to the fall. Keep in mind, however, that in such situations, contributory negligence is hard to prove because the plaintiff can always argue that his or her actions were a result of the medical condition that led to the call (such as a seizure). Also, common law dictates that you take your patients as you find them. Therefore, in some jurisdictions, the patient's actions may not be an adequate defense.

In some states, a successful defense of contributory negligence does not always result in a plaintiff's claim being dismissed outright. Instead, such a defense may lead to a reduction in the damages awarded to the plaintiff based on a **comparative negligence** assessment made by the court.

Gross Negligence and Negligence Per Se

There are some limitations to the use of defenses. These limitations typically arise when the negligence is deemed grossly negligent. **Gross negligence** is a breach that is so offensive that it borders on intentional behavior.

Legally Speaking

immunity Protection from the consequences of litigation; the exemption from being held liable for damages; protection from being sued and having to pay damages; a right of exemption from a duty or penalty.

sovereign immunity Government immunity from negligence liability.

contributory negligence The actions of the plaintiff (the injured person) that fall below the standard to which he should conform for his own protection that may have led, in all or in part, to the harm allegedly caused by the defendant.

comparative negligence The allocation of responsibility for damages to both the plaintiff and defendant based on the relative negligence of the two; the reduction of damages to be recovered by the negligent plaintiff in proportion to his fault.

gross negligence Actions by a defendant that are willful, wanton, or demonstrate a reckless disregard for a duty or standard that result in an injury to the plaintiff.

Legal Practices

Under the theory of negligence, the injury must be directly related to the actions (or lack of actions) of the provider. If the patient dies because of a reason unrelated to the negligent acts of the provider, the provider cannot be found negligent in a court of law—even if the actions in question breached a legal duty of that provider.

Legally Speaking

negligence per se An act or omission that is recognized as negligent as a matter of law because it is contrary to the requirements of the law or because it is so opposed to the dictates of common prudence that one could say, without hesitation or doubt, that no careful person would have committed the act or omission.

cause of action The legal basis for a lawsuit.

Simply stated, gross negligence is inexcusable carelessness or "reckless disregard" that leads to an injury or worsens an already existing illness or injury. For EMS providers, gross negligence occurs when the provider knows or should have known of the detrimental consequences of his or her actions. For example, failure to listen for breath sounds or check for tube placement after intubation may be considered gross negligence. However, keep in mind that whether an action is considered simple or gross negligence is a factual question that is determined by the jury. In the intubation situation, the jury will use the circumstances surrounding the incident to help determine whether failing to check for tube placement was a reckless disregard for the patient's care.

Another form of negligence is **negligence per se.** In this type of negligence, the questions of duty, breach, and causation are eliminated. Generally, this occurs when an individual violates a statute, regulation, or protocol. Some state statutes set forth what violations are considered negligence per se; other classifications of negligence per se originate in case law. In general, in order for an action to be considered negligence per se, such action must be the type of action in which no prudent, reasonable person would partake. In the EMS field, negligence per se most commonly occurs when it is proven that you failed to comply with a statute, your medical protocols, or department policies and procedures. For example, if you show up to work under the influence of illicit drugs or alcohol and you get into a motor vehicle accident with the ambulance or administer the wrong medications, your actions would most likely be considered negligence per se.

Res Ipsa Loquitur

Occasionally, the plaintiff does not have to prove the elements of negligence because the circumstances surrounding the accident and the mere fact that the accident itself occurred raises a legal inference that negligence occurred. In this situation, it is not necessary to prove that the elements of negligence are present. This tactic is known as the legal theory of res ipsa loquitur, which is Latin for "the thing speaks for itself." For example, if an EMT has an extensive history of convictions for driving under the influence and drinking on the job, and that EMT is hired by an ambulance service that did not check his driving record or employment history, and he then kills a patient while on duty because he was driving the ambulance under the influence of alcohol, the case would probably fall into the res ipsa loquitur category.

Unlike gross negligence, in which there still may be questions left for the jury to decide, under a res ipsa loquitur theory, the harm involved is so egregious that a jury trial is normally not necessary. These cases are rare and usually settle out of court quickly.

Causes of Action Under a Negligence Theory

Cause of action is the premise under which the plaintiff brings a lawsuit. There are several causes of action that are applicable to EMS providers, including general and specific claims of negligence such as negligent infliction of emotional distress. As we have discussed, negligence is the most common tort and requires a plaintiff to prove all four elements that show that a breach of the defendant's legal duty caused the plaintiff actual harm.

Negligent infliction of emotional distress is a claim that is usually included in all tort cases. Under this cause of action, the plaintiff states that the defendant's breach not only caused a particular injury, but it also caused emotional distress. In order to successfully recover under this cause of action, physical manifestations of the emotional injury must be offered as evidence. The emotional distress may be proven by a psychiatrist's testimony stating that since the incident the plaintiff (patient) has been depressed, cannot sleep, or has displayed other signs of emotional trauma. Although negligent infliction of emotional distress is usually a claim made in addition to another claim, a plaintiff may use this cause of action as the sole justification of a lawsuit.

Vicarious Liability

Under the legal theory of vicarious liability, liability is shared between the health care provider and his or her employer. This means that your employer, who, by the notion of your employment, has supervision and control over your actions, may be held legally responsible for actions that are committed in the scope of your employment. Further, any person who oversees the services you provide may also be liable. Therefore, not only are you potentially liable for a negligent act, but so is your medical director, your shift supervisor, the owner of the ambulance company, the hospital that provides medical control, and anyone else who has contact with the call and has some form of supervision and control over your actions. Generally, because individual EMS providers have the fewest assets, the plaintiff tries to go after those parties with the greatest assets. Accordingly, lawsuits against individual EMS providers are usually dropped or not initiated at all. It should be noted, however, that both the EMS provider and the EMS agency may be held liable, meaning both may be required to pay damages.

Generally, the theory supporting vicarious liability is that the EMS agency, through its chain of command, has a duty to oversee their individual EMS providers. The lack of such supervision contributes to the breaches that cause injuries. The requirement for oversight may be as broad as providing educational in-services and run reviews or as narrow as requiring that a supervisor appear on certain high-risk calls.

Vicarious liability can be good and bad for the EMS provider. One good aspect is that you are not alone in the suit; other parties, such as the facility for which you work are also involved. However, the involvement of your facility can create a problem. Your employer has more assets to protect than you do, so additional resources are available to protect these assets. This typically means that your employer has the resources to provide legal representation for you when a lawsuit is filed. Unfortunately, if your employer and you are named in the same suit and the same counsel provides representation for both, you may not receive proper legal representation because a conflict of interest may ensue. In certain circumstances, an employer may

Legal Practices

To claim negligent infliction of emotional distress in a civil action, the plaintiff must:

1. Have observed or been the victim of a traumatic event caused by a breach of the defendant's legal duty;
2. Have become emotionally injured because of the observance or occurrence of the traumatic event caused by a breach of the defendant's duty;
3. Manifest physical signs or symptoms of the emotional injury.

benefit from making you look bad and forcing you to take the majority of the blame. Therefore, whenever practical, you should always seek legal representation that is independent from the representation of the department or agency.

Conclusion

Although the primary mission of all EMS providers is to help patients, occasionally accidents occur. In order to compensate patients for the injuries that result from the accident, the legal system has created a form of liability that compensates patients without placing blame or claiming any intentional wrongdoing. You, as a medical provider, have a responsibility to provide care in accordance with the usual and customary manner of other providers under similar circumstances. Failure to act in such a manner is considered a breach of your duties, and can result in personal and department or agency liability for the resulting injury.

Although you cannot always avoid liability or negligent acts, you can minimize your exposure to liability by always following your protocols and treating your patients with respect.

Legal Practices

1. Under the theory of negligence, the injury must be related to the actions, or the failure to act, of the provider. If the patient dies because of a reason unrelated to the negligent acts of the provider, then a causal relationship is not established and the provider cannot be found negligent in a court of law.

2. Providing care that exceeds your scope of practice and training will generally be considered gross negligence. You should never attempt to provide care that exceeds your scope of practice. If, when rendering care, you are unsure whether you should proceed with certain procedures, imagine that your instructor is standing over your shoulder. If you feel that your instructor would fail you for the care you are rendering because it is something that was not covered in your training, you may be liable for gross negligence.

3. When providing care, always contact medical control, and document that medical control was contacted as well as the nature of the discussion. Compliance with these two steps not only ensures that your liability is reduced, but also shares the liability of your actions with the medical director. Remember, as a certified provider, you are working under the medical director's license.

You Be the Judge

Discussion

In order for Jennifer to be found liable for negligence, first, the plaintiff (which would most likely be the patient's family, the patient's estate, or both) would need to prove that Jennifer had a duty to assess the airway after each time they moved the patient. To determine whether or not such duty exists, the plaintiff would refer to the local, regional, and departmental EMS protocols. If airway assessment was required by protocol in this situation, a duty would exist.

The next element of negligence the plaintiff would need to prove is that Jennifer breached this duty. The fact that nothing is mentioned in the patient's chart regarding assessment of the patient's airway does not mean that the airway was not checked. It may simply mean that Jennifer did not document her actions properly, or possibly that the hospital left part of the crew's report out of their chart. However, because the airway assessment is not documented, the assumption of most courts would be that it did not occur. Jennifer would have the burden of proof to show that she did actually assess the patient's airway after moving the patient and during transport. Unless there was someone else in the back of the truck with Jennifer, it would be very difficult for her to prove she did actually perform these assessments. Even if there were someone in the back of the ambulance with Jennifer and the patient, the credibility of that witness would be a question of fact for the jury to determine.

Assuming the plaintiff did prove that Jennifer had a duty to check the airway and that she breached this duty, in order to succeed with a negligence claim the plaintiff would still have to prove that failure to assess the airway directly caused the patient an injury. In this case, the plaintiff has the burden of proving that Jennifer's lack of airway assessment caused the patient's death or prevented the patient from being adequately resuscitated. This would be very difficult for the plaintiff to prove and would undoubtedly involve testimony from several medical experts.

Chapter 8

Intentional Torts

You Be the Judge

You and your partner arrive on-scene at a call in a housing project. The patient is a 2-year-old boy. The parents say that he is sick. You look at the child, and it appears obvious to you that he is very sick. The boy is lethargic and not active. When you ask the parents how long the child has been sick, they give you blank stares. Disgusted by their apparent lack of parenting skills, you simply want to walk away. Trying to get out of there as soon as possible, you suggest that it may be cheaper and easier for the parents to take the child to the local free clinic. After a bit of convincing, the parents agree to take the child to the clinic on their own, but they do not sign an "against medical advice" sheet. When you are back on the road, you make the comment that certain people should not be allowed to have children; your partner agrees. You later hear on the evening news that the child died on a public bus while on the way to the free clinic. Have you committed an intentional tort? If so, for which intentional torts are you liable?

In many lawsuits, issues of liability in negligence are coupled with an intentional tort. An **intentional tort** is an action that the law declares as civilly wrong that is committed by an individual who knowingly intends to commit such an act. This is contrasted with negligence, in which the tortfeasor, the individual who engages in committing the tort, fails to exercise that degree of care in doing what is otherwise permissible.

Types of Intentional Torts

Although the majority of EMS providers do not respond to a call with the intention of causing harm, situations arise in which the EMS provider's lack of restraint, stubbornness, or frustration causes an intentional tort to occur. All intentional torts can be avoided if the provider takes a moment to think about the consequences of his or her actions and knows when those actions may be considered inappropriate. The primary intentional torts are assault, battery, abandonment, false imprisonment, and defamation.

Assault

Assault is defined as any willful attempt to threaten to inflict injury upon another individual, coupled with an apparent present ability to do so, and any intentional display of force that would give the victim reason to fear or expect immediate bodily harm. Assault may be committed without actually touching or doing bodily harm. The act of preparing an IV start kit or drawing up a medication into a syringe in front of a patient who has not consented to your treatment may be considered assault.

ASSAULT: ELEMENTS OF A CAUSE OF ACTION

- Acts intending or perceived to cause a harmful or offensive contact with another.
- An imminent apprehension of such a contact.

Battery

Battery is defined as the unlawful touching of another person. In the case of EMS, a battery may occur despite the good intentions and sincere purpose of providing aid if care is provided without the patient's consent. If consent for treatment is not obtained, a patient can charge you with battery. For example, if an IV is started, or if you strap the patient to the gurney for transport, it is essential that consent be obtained before performing these procedures. The elements of battery are similar to those of assault, but in the case of battery actual physical contact is made to the person without his or her consent.

BATTERY: ELEMENTS OF A CAUSE OF ACTION

- Acts intending to cause a harmful or offensive contact with another person, or an imminent apprehension of such a contact.
- The actual harmful contact or touching without the consent of the person.

Abandonment

A common form of **abandonment** occurs when the EMS provider fails to adequately facilitate a patient transfer. Because EMS providers are not allowed to diagnose patients, they cannot release patients from care. The relationship can only be terminated if (1) the patient is transferred to someone of equal or greater training and certification, or (2) the patient refuses care (even if such a refusal is against medical advice). Accordingly, without standardized protocols that are approved by medical control, a paramedic cannot transfer care of an advanced life support patient to an EMT-Basic.

Proper transfer of care involves a chain of events that starts with a report of the care rendered and the patient's condition and ends with an acknowledgment that the new provider is assuming accountability. Although the acknowledgment does not need to be written, a nurse or physician usually signs an EMS run sheet as evidence of the acceptance of care. Simply transferring a patient from a stretcher onto an emergency department's cot does not fulfill the requirements for a proper transfer of care. Doing so may make an EMS provider liable for abandonment because the patient's care was not handed over to a provider of equal or

Legally Speaking

intentional tort An action, declared to be civilly wrong by the law, that is committed by an individual who knowingly intends to commit such an act.

assault Any willful attempt to threaten to inflict injury upon another individual, coupled with an apparent ability to do so.

battery The unlawful touching of another person. Battery may occur despite good intentions if care is provided without the patient's consent.

abandonment Occurs if a medical provider has entered into a patient-provider relationship, and the medical provider either transfers care to a person of lesser training, does not transfer care to any other provider, or stops providing care for the patient.

greater certification. EMS providers must give information regarding a patient's status directly to the receiving staff. If the staff is not made aware of the patient's condition, it will be much more difficult for them to provide adequate care. Worse yet, without properly notifying the hospital's staff that a new patient was brought in, the hospital staff might not even realize that the patient is waiting to be seen, and the patient could lie for hours unattended.

Another example of abandonment is stopping en route to a call because another event occurred, such as a motor vehicle accident. In such a situation, unless otherwise specified in your local policies, procedures, or protocols, you have a duty to provide care to the original patient for whom you were dispatched. By stopping at a motor vehicle accident to render care, you may have abandoned the first patient that you are already legally committed to treat. Although in most jurisdictions you do not have a legal duty to stop at the scene of a new accident, you do have a duty to call into dispatch and report the new accident so that an available ambulance can be sent if needed.

Although your duty to the first patient may not technically begin until you make actual contact with the patient, the issue is still being debated within the courts. Policies regarding such abandonment vary from jurisdiction to jurisdiction and depend on case law and local protocol. If your protocols do not state otherwise, it is usually most prudent for you to proceed to the original call.

Occasionally, dispatch will reassign you to the new accident scene, particularly if you are the second unit out to the original call or if mutual aid is also responding. If you are reassigned to the motor vehicle accident by dispatch, you should stop to render care to the patients of the accident. Always keep dispatch informed of your actions regarding responses to emergency calls, and always comply with the instructions given to you by dispatch. If you deviate from dispatch's instructions regarding an emergency response for any reason, make sure you inform dispatch, and confirm that dispatch acknowledges you and grants you permission to deviate.

ABANDONMENT: ELEMENTS OF A CAUSE OF ACTION
- Care is sought or needed by a patient.
- A medical provider has entered into a patient-provider relationship with the patient (such relationship should be assumed to commence as soon as the EMS provider acknowledges the call for service).
- The medical provider transfers care to a person of lesser training, or does not transfer care to any other provider.
- The medical provider stops providing care for the patient while the patient still requires care.

Many departments have implemented a staged response system. In this system, different types of providers are dispatched according to proper protocols and the rapid identification of illnesses or injuries that require advanced care. This system, however, may give rise to an abandonment situation. For example, if a paramedic arrives on the scene and establishes patient contact, it is legally risky for that provider to leave the scene before the basic life support (BLS) unit arrives, even if the nature of the call to which the paramedic responded is basic. The paramedic must remain on the scene and take adequate measures to determine that the patient does not require any advanced life support intervention.

Even if the BLS unit is on scene, transferring care to that unit could be considered abandonment if the patient requires paramedic level advanced life support services. A sprained ankle with syncopal episode may really disguise an arrhythmia-induced syncopal episode with the associated fall. Only too late, after detriment to the patient, would it be discovered that the paramedic should have continued to care for the patient and not have abandoned the scene by turning care over to the lesser trained and equipped BLS crew. Similarly, if a BLS unit calls for advanced life support, the EMTs must remain with the patient until the paramedics arrive and acknowledge that they are assuming patient care.

A thorough medical evaluation of the patient assists in eliminating the risk of patient abandonment. You should contact your local medical director, system administrator, or legal counsel to determine how the tort of abandonment affects your actions as an EMS provider in a dual-staged or multi-tiered system.

Legally Speaking

false imprisonment The nonconsensual, intentional confinement of a person.

False Imprisonment

If a competent patient requests to be released from medical care or refuses to receive the care you are offering, you must honor the patient's wishes. If you ignore the patient's wishes and take the patient to the hospital despite his or her request, you may be liable for **false imprisonment.**

FALSE IMPRISONMENT: ELEMENTS OF A CAUSE OF ACTION

- The nonconsensual, intentional confinement of a person.
- Confinement occurs without lawful privilege (that is, there is no factor present, such as mental incapacitation, that would allow the patient to be confined against his or her will).
- Confinement lasts for an appreciable period of time.

An example of a situation that may lead to a false imprisonment claim is if a patient has a syncopal episode that is relieved upon arrival by the EMS unit, and the patient is transported without providing consent. Many times, patients have a history of syncope that proves to have no medical explanation of its origin after thorough medical testing. When future episodes occur, these patients frequently request to not be transported to the hospital. If you disobey the patient's wishes to be released, you may be liable for the tort of false imprisonment. This scenario occurred in *Cathey v. City of Louisville,* a case heard by the Kentucky Court of Appeals in 1999. In this case, a 19-year-old woman was found unconscious while working as a housekeeper in a Louisville hotel. When the paramedics arrived, the patient was awake and hysterical. Her blood pressure was low and her respiratory rate was high. However, the patient refused transport to the hospital. The paramedics on-scene ignored her request, and, with the help of a police officer, restrained her and transported her to a hospital. The patient sued for false imprisonment and battery. In this situation, statutory and sovereign immunity were not enough to protect the EMS providers from liability for false imprisonment.

Legally Speaking

defamation The spoken or written falsehood by a defendant about a plaintiff that causes damage to the plaintiff's reputation or standing within the community; the publication of anything that injures the good name or reputation of another or brings him or her into disrepute.

slander The spoken form of defamation.

libel The written form of defamation.

False imprisonment may occur without the application of physical restraints. Simply refusing to allow a patient to terminate care may be considered false imprisonment. This is where using the legal ABCs (presented in Chapter 3) may be beneficial. By documenting the patient's responses as well as respecting the patient's wishes, it is less likely that the patient will allege that you held him or her against his or her will.

A common scenario that can be incorrectly construed as false imprisonment is when a patient who is suffering from a narcotic overdose receives a narcotic antagonist to reverse the effects of the overdose. After the antagonist is administered, the patient may seem competent. At this time, the patient typically becomes upset and requests to be released. Such patients commonly threaten a lawsuit for false imprisonment if you proceed to take them to the hospital against their will. This is a controversial scenario because the antagonist has a short half-life and is likely to wear off in 15 to 30 minutes, thus returning the patient to the previous overdose status. Because the patient's competence is considered only temporary, transporting him or her to the hospital usually does not fall within the confines of false imprisonment.

Defamation

Information released to the public that is not true may give rise to liability under the legal theory of defamation of character. **Defamation** is the spoken or written falsehood about another person that results in damage to that person's reputation or standing within the community. Spoken defamation is known as **slander.** For instance, if you are in any type of public forum and you describe a coworker as a drunk, you may be liable for defamation. Written falsehoods are known as **libel.**

Defamatory actions are not limited to the intentional spreading of falsehoods about an individual. These actions may also be against another fire department, ambulance service, hospital, or health organization. Keep in mind that it is much better to handle internal or interagency disputes through the appropriate channels rather than risk subjection to the unnecessary and burdensome litigation of a libel or slander suit.

Slander and libel have not been common in the field of EMS; however, this may change. One event that may cause this intentional tort is the disclosure of confidential information. For instance, in today's society in which certain illnesses, such as acquired immunodeficiency syndrome (AIDS), may lead to discrimination, public disclosure of a patient's condition may be detrimental to the patient. If you disclose such confidential information, you may be liable for libel and slander (if the information is proven to not be completely accurate), the intentional tort of invasion of privacy, and state and federal civil and criminal penalties for the disclosure of protected health care information.

LIBEL AND SLANDER: ELEMENTS OF A CAUSE OF ACTION

- Libel consists of the publication of defamatory matter by written or printed words, by its embodiment in physical form, or by any other form of communication that has a potentially harmful and unjust characteristic.

- Slander consists of the publication of defamatory matter by spoken words, transitory gestures, or any form of communication other than those stated in the definition of libel.

Punitive Damages

Punitive damages are monetary rewards awarded by courts in an effort to punish wrongdoers in civil actions involving intentional torts or to dissuade a party from future intentional behavior that is detrimental to the public. Punitive damages are often used to punish repetitive behavior that is intentional and tortuous in nature. In some cases, gross negligence may also warrant the application of an additional monetary award.

Punitive damages are assessed beyond the amount necessary to compensate for an individual's injuries. The amount allowed for punitive damages varies in different jurisdictions, but may be as much as millions of dollars. The amount of punitive damages assessed is not related to the extent of the injury, but more the nature of the wrongful act committed.

Legally Speaking

punitive damages Monetary rewards awarded by courts in an effort to punish wrongdoers in civil actions involving intentional torts, or to dissuade a party from future intentional behavior that is detrimental to the public.

Legal Practices

1. The best way to protect yourself from any intentional tort claim is to document the reasons for your actions. Documentation of items, such as the patient's provision of consent and to what they consented, commonly negates an assault or battery charge.

2. There are only two times when an EMT is allowed to leave a patient: (a) when another health care provider with an equal or greater scope of practice assumes care and signs a form acknowledging such an assumption of care, or (b) the patient refuses care *and* signs a form acknowledging such refusal. In either case, as the treating EMT you must document how and why your treatment of the patient stopped, whether the patient was transferred, and to whom the care was transferred.

3. Informal public discussion about various patients may be considered defamation—especially in small towns or communities where providers know the patients. Despite your best clinical judgment, you may not always know for sure whether a person has a particular condition or diagnosis. Publicly discussing with fellow colleagues a diagnosis about a patient whom everyone knows, especially when the diagnosis is wrong, is not only a violation of patient confidentiality, but is also defamation. Therefore, do not tell "war stories" when the identity of the patient can be figured out by others in the discussion.

Conclusion

Intentional torts are not only detrimental to the EMS provider personally, but may serve to destroy the morale of the entire department or agency. When one commits an intentional tort, any respect that is held for the provider and the provider's agency is destroyed. The patient is personally offended and is likely to seek retribution and retaliation. This may come in the form of publicity and a lawsuit. The publicity may lead to public outrage, leading to decreased public approval. This may eventually translate into diminished financial resources being generated from the public via tax dollars or donations because the bad publicity would likely make the public unwilling to vote for or financially support initiatives that support "questionable" EMS services.

These acts may be avoided by maintaining a cool head and thinking before one acts. Following the legal ABCs (always documenting thoroughly, being kind to the patient, and contacting medical control) may help you avoid the consequences that arise from intentional torts.

You Be the Judge

Discussion

At a minimum, in this case, you would be liable for abandonment. A review of the elements of abandonment in relation to these facts show that defending an abandonment claim under these circumstances would most likely be futile:

1. *Care is sought or needed by a patient.* Care was sought as soon as 9-1-1 was called and EMS was requested.

2. *A medical provider has entered into a patient-provider relationship with the patient.* As soon as you made contact with the child and his parents, a patient-provider relationship was established.

3. *The medical provider transfers care to a person of lesser training or does not transfer care to any other provider.* In this case, you left the child in the care of the parents, who, in your own estimation, were unfit to adequately care for the child.

4. *The medical provider stops providing care for the patient.* By leaving the patient without transporting him to a hospital, you stopped providing care.

5. *The patient still requires care.* The fact that the child died illustrates that he still required care. However, even if the child did not die, your own assessment concluded that the child was lethargic and inactive— symptoms of a potentially serious ailment. Furthermore, the parents did not sign a refusal sheet, which shows that they felt the child needed further medical treatment.

In addition to the abandonment claim, if your comment that certain people should not be allowed to have children was stated publicly, heard by others, and ultimately construed as damaging to the reputation of the boy's parents, you may also be liable for defamation.

Bibliography

Cathey v. City of Louisville Ky. App. LEXIS 108 (1999).

Chapter 9

Criminal Violations

You Be the Judge

You are working your third shift for a private ambulance company. As a part of your employment you sometimes serve as stand-by medical coverage at car races and sporting events. After a particularly boring day at an auto race, your partner, a senior medic with the service, breaks out the ice chest. He reveals that he has a false bottom in the chest, and in the secret compartment he happens to have a six-pack of beer. Although the race is over, you cannot leave for the next two hours, until all of the racing teams have left. Your partner suggests that it is fine to have a few drinks, because there is little chance that anyone will need your services. Trusting his judgment because he is a senior medic, you decide to drink a beer with him. Forty-five minutes after you start drinking, you are called to respond to the pits to help a crew member who dropped an engine on his foot. En route, you plow your ambulance into the star racing team's trailer and total their prize car. What is your liability?

Case Study

State v. Montecalvo (1990) Ohio App. LEXIS 3942
Michael Montecalvo was a certified paramedic in the state of Ohio. While driving an ambulance in response to an emergency call, Montecalvo drove through a red light and struck an automobile at an intersection. Montecalvo and his partner were not injured; however, the driver of the other automobile, who was pregnant at the time, died as a result of the accident. Montecalvo was indicted on six separate counts, including aggravated vehicular homicide, involuntary manslaughter, and reckless operation of an emergency vehicle.

The jury found the paramedic not guilty of aggravated vehicular homicide; however, they did find the paramedic guilty of involuntary manslaughter and failing to proceed with due regard in an emergency vehicle past a red signal.

The *Montecalvo* case caused an uproar in the EMS community in the early 1990s. Montecalvo previously had a stellar history in EMS with many years of dedicated service. After this case, Montecalvo's certification was revoked, and he was fined and imprisoned.

Unfortunately, the occurrence of EMS providers committing traffic violations is on the rise. EMS providers are not immune from the ramifications of violating traffic or criminal laws. Every state has traffic laws dictating the operation of an emergency vehicle. Although some states are less stringent than others, no state law gives any emergency vehicle operator the right to drive recklessly or without regard for the safety of other persons using the streets or highways. The EMS oath of "do no harm" should inspire EMS providers to recognize that they are of little help to patients if they fail to arrive on the scene or at the hospital because of an accident caused by reckless driving.

Being indicted or arrested on a criminal charge can be one of the scariest moments of your life. Understanding the criminal process may not only alleviate some of the mystery involved with the process, but will provide you with a basic understanding of your rights as an American citizen if you become entangled in the criminal justice system. Above all, the criminal system is designed to determine beyond a reasonable doubt the guilt of an accused. Whereas punishment and retribution are also roles of the criminal system, this chapter addresses the criminal system's process of determining guilt, including the trial and related proceedings as well as different types of criminal liability to which EMS providers may be exposed.

The Criminal System

There are different roles within the criminal system. Each role has a specific responsibility and set of duties within the system.

- **The police** are a quasi-military agency. They are part of the executive branch of the government. Each municipality has the jurisdictional power to create and operate a police force. Under the guidance of state and federal laws and the U.S. Constitution, the police are provided certain powers that extend beyond the rights of a normal citizen. These additional powers serve to protect citizens and uphold and enforce the law. The police are responsible for arresting suspected criminals and collecting evidence.
- **The district attorney or prosecutor** is an attorney who acts on behalf of the state or federal government and the citizens. The prosecutor is responsible for using the evidence against a suspect to create a case that proves beyond a reasonable doubt that the suspect is guilty of the crime.
- **The defense attorney** is an attorney who represents the rights and interests of the accused. Access to a defense attorney is a right that all accused are granted even if they cannot afford to pay for the legal services provided. The defense attorney is responsible for showing that a doubt may exist as to whether the accused is guilty.
- **The grand jury** is composed of a group of citizens who are randomly selected and assigned to a confidential forum during

which preliminary matters regarding the substance of the prosecutor's case are presented. The grand jury is responsible for hearing evidence presented by the prosecutor and determining, based on this evidence, whether probable cause exists, allowing the accused to continue to be held for trial. The grand jury makes this determination through the use of an indictment, a legal determination that there is enough evidence against an accused to support a trial.

■ **The jury** is a group of citizens responsible for determining factual issues in a case. Unlike the grand jury, this jury determines the actual guilt or innocence of the accused, not just whether the state has probable cause to pursue charges for a crime. The right to have a case heard before a jury is guaranteed in the U.S. Constitution.

■ **The judge** is responsible for ensuring that the legal process operates smoothly and orderly with minimal complications. The judge is responsible for determining all questions of law or legal issues.

The criminal system proceeds differently depending on whether the crime is a felony or misdemeanor. Misdemeanors are crimes that are not as serious as felonies. Penalties for misdemeanors may only involve fines or limited prison time. A misdemeanor offense may not stay on your permanent record, and generally employers, as well as other public entities, are not entitled to learn of misdemeanor convictions. Examples of misdemeanors include shoplifting merchandise valued under a specified amount and trespassing. In some states, violating certain EMS regulations, such as practicing as an EMT without being properly certified, may be a misdemeanor.

In most instances, police do not have the authority to arrest you for a misdemeanor if they did not see you commit the act. However, if you commit a misdemeanor act in front of a police officer, you may be arrested. If someone files a complaint alleging that you may have committed a misdemeanor, a citation may be written or a warrant may be ordered for your arrest. You may have to go to the police station to answer questions and file a counter-report, or you may be arraigned immediately for the crime in front of a judge.

Felonies are considered serious crimes. They may be violent, such as murder, attempted murder, or rape. They may also be nonviolent, such as drug trafficking, embezzling, or tax evasion. Felony convictions typically result in incarceration. A felony record is public information and future employers have a right to access your past felony record.

You may be arrested for a felony even if you did not commit the felony in front of a police officer. Depending on the circumstances, police officers have the authority to arrest you when they have probable cause that you recently committed a felony—even if the act did not occur in their presence. If the district attorney or federal prosecutor feels there is probable cause that you committed a felony, a warrant may be issued for your arrest. In some jurisdictions, a grand jury indictment may be required before a warrant may be issued.

After you are arrested, you are held in jail until the preliminary hearing. Matters such as motions to dismiss evidence, bail, and informing you of your rights and the charges against you are handled during the preliminary hearing. If there is evidence that may not have been properly obtained or if there is ample evidence that an individual's constitutional rights have been violated, the defense attorney addresses these issues during the preliminary hearing by requesting that improperly obtained evidence be disregarded or the charges be dismissed.

After the preliminary hearing, both sides prepare their case. Interviews may be conducted or additional evidence may be gathered. If you have not made bail, you may be in jail during this entire time. This may last as long as six months, depending on the requirements of your jurisdiction.

At the trial, the prosecutor presents the state's case. Your defense attorney then presents your case. The sole function of the first phase of the trial is to determine guilt. The jury is asked to determine beyond a reasonable doubt whether you are guilty. If you are found guilty, the trial moves into the sentencing phase. This part of the trial may also involve the presentation of evidence and testimony. The jury or the judge may then determine the length of your sentence.

If you are determined to be not guilty, you are released and the charges are dropped. Unlike your right to appeal, the state is not allowed to retry you on the same charges. However, if the jury cannot answer the question and the jury results in a hung trial, the proceedings may begin all over again, and you could be tried as if the first trial never happened. A hung jury results when the jury's vote for a verdict ends in a tie or, in a case such as a felony criminal charge where a unanimous verdict is required, a verdict is not reached.

If you are found guilty, you may appeal. An appeal consists of an argument regarding the procedure of the criminal process. You cannot appeal a jury's determination of fact, but you can appeal a judge's determination of law. For example, if the jury determines that you hit your patient, this determination of fact cannot be appealed. However, you may appeal the judge's instructions to the jury regarding the legal theory of self-defense and how such theory should have been applied to the facts of the case. An appeal may affect the jury's findings of the facts, which means that the results of the old trial are required to be dismissed and the prosecutor must retry the government's case against you. For example, if your attorney objects to the inclusion of a piece of evidence and that objection is overruled, but the jury uses the evidence in the process of determining guilt, you may appeal that the decision by the judge to overrule the objection was wrong. As a result of that wrong decision, the jury heard evidence that they should not have, and thus, they may have made a wrong finding.

Types of Criminal Liability

EMS providers have the potential to incur various types of criminal liability. These criminal liabilities include driving violations and subsequent crimes, criminal violation of narcotics and controlled substance laws, criminal assault and battery, theft, desecration of a corpse, sexual misconduct, as well as various fraud and abuse violations.

Responding to a scene with flashing lights and sirens activated does not allow an EMS provider to drive recklessly. Many studies have shown that responding with lights and sirens on does not save a significant amount of time when compared to responding without lights and sirens. Many states even have laws that regulate how you are to operate an emergency vehicle. Reckless disregard for driving safety may cause criminal liability for violating the traffic laws. Further, should you be involved in a motor vehicle collision as a result of violating these laws, you may be liable for the consequences, including vehicular manslaughter.

Criminal assault and battery charges result from blatant disregard for a patient's rights. Striking or forcibly restraining a patient or reckless care that is provided against the express wishes of a competent patient may be considered criminal assault and battery. Medicine is sometimes referred to "as the practice of legalized assault and battery" because without the consent of a patient, you may be liable for assault and battery in criminal as well as civil suits.

Theft is another serious offense for EMS providers. Theft is the unlawful taking of a person's possessions without his or her permission. Theft can be classified as a misdemeanor or a felony depending on the amount that is taken. There are old jokes about how the first thing an EMS provider checks is the patient's wallet or that the "C" in the legal ABCs stands for cash. These jokes are inappropriate, but they exist because of past actions of some dishonorable EMS providers.

Desecration of a corpse occurs when one performs inappropriate actions on the dead. Although EMS providers, for the most part, do not intentionally act with this type of criminal activity in mind, EMTs have been charged with this crime. For example, it was discovered that providers were practicing intubation techniques and other invasive clinical skills on an obviously expired patient. In the past, such actions may have been considered acceptable practice in emergency medicine, but today they are considered ethically wrong, and criminal charges may be levied. Should a family member or fellow health care provider report an EMT's involvement in these types of acts, prosecution under the desecration of a corpse laws may ensue.

Sexual misconduct is a serious concern in the modern health care industry. Respecting your patient and your patient's rights is the best protection against this form of criminal liability. Further protection may include the use of three-person crews, so that the patient is never left alone with one provider. Female providers should be considered to provide care for female patients who may be victims of sexual assault or have a history of psychiatric problems that leads them to being paranoid, delusional, or accusatory.

Finally, as discussed later in Chapters 12 and 13, a felony offense may arise from nonclinical actions. Violations through civil rights claims or fraud and abuse claims may subject you to criminal liability. Familiarity with these laws may prevent or reduce your liability.

Legal Practices

When valuables are taken away from a patient, you should document what was removed, where and how the items were stored, and to whom the items were given upon arrival to the emergency department. Creating a record of the patient's valuables may reduce the risk of potential criminal and civil liability.

Implications of a Felony Offense

A felony offense can result in loss of freedom through incarceration and, perhaps, financial penalties through fines. In addition, a felony offense may lead to the revocation of your certification to function as an EMS provider in most states. It may also interfere with your ability to gain lawful employment upon release from prison. Finally, the professional reputation and respect that you may have worked hard to earn from your colleagues will likely be destroyed.

Conclusion

Although criminal liability is not a common occurrence in the field of EMS, EMS providers are not immune. Should you be accused of any criminal act, you should seek an attorney immediately. This is a complicated and daunting process that will be extremely stressful. The best advice that you can follow is to familiarize yourself with the criminal laws of your jurisdiction, and always act in an appropriate, professional manner, even including driving to an emergency call.

Legal Practices

1. If arrested or taken into police custody, the best way to protect yourself is by not talking without your attorney present. Once you ask for your attorney to be present, the police cannot continue with their interrogation until your attorney arrives. You must be the one asking for the attorney, however. If your attorney shows up and you have not asked for him or her, they do not have the right to stop or join in the interrogation.

2. Unlike your home or personal property, the government has a right, through its police powers, to search your ambulance without a warrant. As a regulated industry, health care organizations have waived the right to require a warrant for searches. If you are stopped, you should cooperate with the government official as soon as you have reasonable evidence that the person is legitimate.

You Be the Judge

Discussion

In this scenario, you would be liable under a gross negligence theory for any damages to the racing team's property. You would also be liable under a gross negligence theory to the patient with the foot injury if the delay in response, treatment, and transport caused by your accident resulted in identifiable harm to the patient.

Under these circumstances, drinking while on duty is so contrary to readily accepted public policy that you would most likely be liable for punitive damages as well as actual damages. You would also probably be liable to your employer for any of the damage to the ambulance or other equipment caused by your recklessness. Administratively, these actions would likely cause you to have your license or certification to practice revoked.

Finally, depending on the specific laws of your state involving driving under the influence, having an open container of alcohol in a motor vehicle, and being involved in an motor vehicle accident while drinking or under the influence, it is very likely that you would be liable for a criminal offense. Being convicted for such offenses may lead to permanent or temporary loss of your driver's license, civil fines, and incarceration.

Bibliography

State v. Montecalvo 1990 Ohio App. LEXIS 3942 (1990).

Chapter 10

Due Process and Disciplinary Procedures

You Be the Judge

You receive a letter from the state that revokes your EMT certification. You respond in writing asking for justification for the revocation. The state does not respond. A friend who has a friend that works for the state says that she heard that comments you made at a recent advisory meeting upset a state employee and that the employee revoked your certification to get even. Can you continue to work as an EMT under the theory that the revocation was unjustified?

As an American citizen, you have certain inalienable rights. The source of these freedoms is stated clearly in the Constitution of the United States: "Under God, all men are created equal . . . endowed with inalienable rights . . . the right to life, liberty, and the pursuit of happiness." Over the years, courts have interpreted this phrase to mean that from these rights other rights are derived. For example, based on this phrase, courts have upheld an individual's right to refuse lifesaving medical care and the right to privacy in family-planning matters. You also have certain rights when it comes to property, employment, and education. In addition, you have rights that protect you against discrimination, persecution, and slavery. All of these rights are provided to American citizens by the Constitution.

What rights do you have as an EMS provider? This is an important question that is very closely related to the type of accreditation that your state has provided. While the debate of licensure versus certification is ongoing, it does have a practical legal implication. Attorney, EMS expert, former paramedic, and publisher of the *Journal of Emergency Medical Services (JEMS)*, James O. Page suggests in his October 1999 *JEMS* article, "Whose License is it Anyway?" that the difference between licensure and certification is the basis for determining the level of due process that an EMS provider is entitled to receive in administrative disciplinary matters.

EMS and Due Process

The first question that must be answered is whether every health care provider is afforded due process with respect to employment disciplinary matters. Due process is the right to be treated in a fair, objective, non-biased manner. The Fourteenth Amendment of the U.S. Constitution prohibits any state or local government from depriving any person of life, liberty, or property without the due process of the law.

Does a certification or licensure relate to life, liberty, and property? The courts have determined that an individual's employment is considered property. In the 1972 case *Board of Regents of State Colleges v. Roth,* the United States Supreme Court held that "to have a property interest in [an employment] benefit, a person clearly must have more than an abstract need or desire for it. He must have more than a unilateral expectation of it. He must, instead, have a legitimate claim of entitlement to it." Further, the Supreme Court reiterated that without procedural due process an employee cannot be deprived of any constitutionally protected property right. Shifting from the topic of benefits to the topic of mere employment, in 1985, the Supreme Court stated in *Cleveland Bd. of Educ. v. Loudermill* that certain public employees have property rights, and that termination or alteration of the terms of their employment without due process is prohibited.

Because the majority of states have a statutory requirement for retaining a certification or licensure, a link exists between your certification and the state. Accordingly, you, as a provider, have a property interest in your certification because you are only able to maintain employment with a valid certification. The courts have further held that even in the absence of a statutory requirement, a local law, contract, or administrative regulation regarding an occupation in the public sector provides the necessary justification for the property interest. Thus, all governmental EMS agencies, either expressly or implied through contract, have a duty to provide due process to its employees when dealing with disciplinary matters.

Does a private employer also have a due process requirement? Since 1980, there have been numerous decisions affirming such a notion. The California courts have been the forerunner in answering "yes" to this question. The affirmative court rulings have been based upon theories ranging from estoppel (good-faith reliance) to an implied contract. The theory of estoppel would hold that an employee provides labor and talent to the employer in return for a salary and the reasonable expectation that he or she will be treated fairly in employment matters. Such theory "estopps" an employer from claiming the employment-at-will defense (that the employer can fire an employee for any reason) when faced with claims regarding unfair treatment in promotions or termination. Further, because most private EMS companies function in certain capacities as an extension of the legal and operational branches of the government through municipal contracting, they may, depending on the jurisdiction, be required to provide their employees with the same rights as the governmental agency would be required to provide when functioning on behalf of the government.

What Is Due Process?

In trying to define what due process is, the courts have suggested that it means "fundamental fairness and substantial justice." (For example, see the 1938 case *Morgan v. United States.*) In most cases, this means that an employee has a right to have an administrative hearing when any disciplinary action is taken that impacts his or her certification or licensure. An administrative hearing, unlike a judicial hearing, usually does not occur in a courtroom. Administrative hearings are held in various settings. At an administrative hearing, a fair and unbiased mediator, administrative law judge, board, or commission listens to the circumstances of the disciplinary action and the evidence that is presented for and against you, and then decides based on that state's administrative law rules and procedures if the disciplinary action you received was fair and substantiated.

How Does Due Process Work?

In those states that have adopted licensure for paramedics, the paramedic enjoys more rights and a more intimate relationship with the state. Depending on the state's licensing authority, a licensed paramedic may also enjoy certain privileges that their certified counterparts may not have, such as performing medical procedures without direct supervision of medical control. When a state attempts to revoke a paramedic's license, it results in a lengthy and expensive—but fair—process, similar to that of a physician. Unlike states in which a paramedic is merely certified, in a state where a paramedic holds a license, a license or permission to practice cannot be revoked unless a formal hearing is held with the state's licensure board. With this process in place, licensed paramedics may avoid the unfair and illegal actions that may occur without the protection of full due process.

Jurisdictions where EMS providers are certified rather than licensed are less likely to provide such formal hearing and appeal rights regarding professional discipline. As stated previously, almost all EMS providers are entitled to due process when disciplinary actions ensue; however, there are occasions in which local systems that use certified EMS providers take advantage of the naivety of those providers who are not in a position to understand the administrative law system or cannot afford an attorney skilled enough to resolve the complications that arise during such proceedings. In such situations, the local medical director or the local EMS agency simply disregards, or inconsistently applies, due process requirements for certified providers. Furthermore, because very few providers understand the due process rights that a certified provider is actually entitled to, documentation of the process of certification revocation or suspension is rare.

Baxter v. Fulton-DeKalb Hospital Authority is a good example of a case in which a federal court held that a paramedic (who was certified, not licensed) did have a valid claim for violation of due process. The paramedic's local medical director revoked his right to practice without a hearing. Although the paramedic was cleared of any misconduct by a hospital investigation, the medical director, who was employed by a public hospital, refused to allow the paramedic to return to his position. The paramedic successfully sued, claiming violation of due process because he was not afforded the rights to which he was entitled.

Specific Due Process Provisions

California is one example of a state that uses licensure for paramedics rather than certification. In fact, it was the first state in the nation to alter its legislation to provide for licensure. In its state codes (CA Codes § 1797.194 and CA Codes § 1797.100), California made the EMS authority a division of the Health and Welfare Agency. This agency has a multitude of powers and responsibilities, including that of licensing paramedics, defining their scope of practice, and overseeing disciplinary procedures. California Code § 1797.194(d) provides that all disciplinary proceedings are to be conducted in accordance with Part 1 of Division 3 of Title 2 of the Code, a section that calls for judicial oversight for disciplinary procedures.

Some states have established formal due process legislation for EMS providers regardless of whether the providers are certified or licensed. In these states, the general administrative procedure statutes provide for administrative hearings when any actions may interfere with a provider's ability to practice. The format and venue of the hearings are set forth in the state's code.

Table 10.1 shows the due process provisions for accredited personnel for each state. Twenty-six states do not provide any guidance for disciplinary actions or due process. Eighteen states describe their grounds for disciplinary actions and their process for how such actions are undertaken. Four states merely give the grounds; two provide the statutory right to due process.

Problems with Due Process

The largest problem EMS providers face with due process requirements is the ease with which EMS systems can avoid adhering to the requirements without EMS providers knowing that their rights have been violated.

The fact that the terms of the certification require oversight from a medical director is the primary reason why rights violations occur. For example, in some systems, the medical director is given the power to circumvent any valid disciplinary process that has been established. This means that the medical director can pretty much fire or discipline an EMS provider at will. This is an undocumented aspect of the EMS practice environment. As another example, Ohio's Division of EMS has an appeals process that has been established to address issues of disciplinary actions involving the EMS provider's certification status. However, because the majority of the disciplinary actions are handled within an EMS department, the state rarely has a need to formally investigate an EMS provider or use the appeals process.

Table 10.1

Due Process Provisions by State

State	Provision for due process in disciplinary procedures
AL	N
AK	N
AZ	GR; DP
AR	N
CA	N
CO	N
CT	DP
DE	GR; DP
DC	N
FL	GR
GA	GR; DP
HI	GR; DP
ID	N
IL	GR; DP
IN	GR
IA	GR; DP
KS	GR; DP
KY	N
LA	GR
ME	GR; DP
MD	GR; DP
MA	N
MI	GR; DP
MN	GR; DP
MO	GR; DP
MS	N
MT	N
NE	GR
NV	N
NH	GR
NM	N
NJ	N
NY	N
NC	N
ND	N
OH	N
OK	N
OR	GR; DP
PA	GR; DP
RI	N
SC	N
SD	N
TN	GR; DP
TX	GR; DP
UT	GR; DP
VT	N
VA	N
WA	DP
WV	GR; DP
WI	N
WY	N

Key: GR = Grounds that due process procedures can be evoked; DP = Due process procedure; N = Not mentioned

The following case study illustrates this problem:

A man was a career fire fighter and paramedic in one city and the volunteer fire chief in a neighboring jurisdiction. While he was on duty at the volunteer station, a call came in requesting assistance for a patient complaining of difficulty breathing. The primary ambulance crew was out on another call, so the paramedic took another fire fighter with him and responded to the call in the secondary ambulance. The paramedic assessed the patient and began an initial treatment regimen. The paramedic then had to wait over 40 minutes for the primary crew to show up and transport the patient. Rather than wait for the primary crew, the patient (who was stable at the time) was loaded into the ambulance and transported to the hospital across the street. The paramedic sat in the back of the ambulance with the patient. The fire fighter drove.

As a result of these actions, the paramedic was suspended by local medical control for allegedly violating a state law by transporting a patient in an ambulance staffed with only one certified EMT. The medical director of the EMS agency that the paramedic worked for was able to impose a suspension from work without any involvement of the state. Although the suspension resulted from actions that the paramedic performed while working for the volunteer department, the suspension also applied to his career job because that facility used the same physician as its medical director. Upon request from the paramedic's attorney, the hospital that provided the medical control did finally allow the paramedic a hearing. The hearing resulted in an elimination of the suspension, and the paramedic was able to regain employment. Without the persistence of the paramedic's attorney in requesting a hearing, however, the paramedic's suspension most likely would not have been lifted.

What Can You Do?

First, know your rights. As long as you are certified or licensed by the state, you have a right to due process for any disciplinary matter in which you are involved that may result in action such as suspension or revocation of your state licensure or certification. Accordingly, your employer cannot fire, suspend, or revoke your right to practice without a hearing, unless specifically allowed under state law or contract.

Second, if you are accused of a violation of a policy, procedure, or something else, use these tips to protect yourself:

- Request that any and all accusations be substantiated in writing immediately.
- Request a meeting with a supervisor and your medical director to discuss the accusation.
- Take someone that is on your side with you to the meeting. According to the National Labor Relations Board, you have a right, regardless if you are union or not, to have a person of your choice at all disciplinary meetings or hearings. Bringing your lawyer to the meeting helps ensure that your employer focuses on providing you with due process.
- Document your side of the matter in writing. Keep a copy for yourself and submit a copy to your employer.

Legal Practices

1. Familiarize yourself with the protocols, policies, and expectations of your medical director. Understanding the acceptable practices and standards of your medical director will help you establish a rapport and allow you to demonstrate your skills and abilities as an EMS provider.

2. Make sure that you have a recent copy of your state's EMS laws and regulations and the state's administrative law practice acts or equivalent. These commonly provide guidelines for due process and disciplinary hearings.

- If, after the meeting, you feel that your certification or license is being unfairly revoked or suspended, obtain an attorney.
- Notify the state immediately of this violation of your due process.

Conclusion

As a state-recognized medical provider, you have a right to due process regarding any matter that affects your ability to practice within your accredited level of licensure or certification. This right can trace its origins to the Constitution. Knowing your due process rights can protect you if you are ever accused of any wrongdoing. Exercising your rights is essential in maintaining and preserving your rights to a fair and just work environment.

You Be the Judge

Discussion

You certainly cannot continue to work if your certification has been revoked. Regardless of how procedurally improper the proceedings may have been regarding your revocation, any revocation by a duly authorized state agency is recognized as enforceable by the courts until such time the revocation is reversed by either the state agency or a court. If you do practice under such conditions, even if your revocation is already on appeal, you face the risk of violating the law that prohibits practice without certification, and those actions may even lead to criminal penalties such as fines and incarceration.

If your certification was revoked in what you believe was an improper manner, you should first research the administrative disciplinary procedural statutes or regulations of your state. You should then take advantage of whatever appeal process is afforded to you by that statute or regulation. Many states have a provision in their administrative disciplinary statutes allowing for direct appeal to an upper-level state court from any decision adverse to the licensed or certified provider. You may need the services of an attorney to assist you with the appeals process. If after all of your appeals are exhausted and you still have not prevailed and your attorney feels you have a strong case, you may attempt to sue the state in federal court for violation of your state and constitutional right to due process.

Bibliography

Baxter v. Fulton-DeKalb Hospital Authority, 764 F.S. 1510 (1991).

Board of Regents of State Colleges v. Roth, 408 U.S. 564, 577 (1972).

Cleveland Bd. of Educ. v. Loudermill, 470 U.S. 532 (1985).

Morgan v. United States, 304 U.S. 1, 18–19 (1938).

Page, James O. "Whose License is it Anyway?" *Journal of Emergency Medical Services* (October 1999).

Documentation

You Be the Judge

You have just finished intubating a patient. You document the time that you intubated and the fact that you heard equal bilateral breath sounds upon auscultation. You write these notes on a piece of tape that you stick to the side of your pants. You plan on transferring the information to the patient care report (PCR) later. During the transport, the tape falls off of your leg before you are able to transfer the information to the PCR. Because you lost the tape, you never transfer the information to the written report. Upon arrival at the emergency department, the endotracheal tube is dislodged. Your PCR does not indicate that you assessed your intubation for accuracy or patency. Two years later you are named in a lawsuit for wrongful death. How will you prove that you successfully intubated the patient? What is your liability?

Just as airway is the most important part of any EMS clinical course, documentation is the single most important item in an EMS law course. The quality of your documentation can either create liability or protect you. Therefore, EMS professionals should always remember and abide by the following rule:

Always document. If you did not document it, you did not do it!

This chapter discusses the benefits of documentation and addresses the do's and don'ts of documentation. By applying the principles described in this chapter, you can help reduce the risk of liability you encounter working in the field.

Basics of Documentation

The medical record is an invaluable clinical resource and perhaps the most important component of the continuum of care that patients rely on throughout the course of treatment. Every provider who has any patient contact uses the medical record. The medical record is utilized for tasks, such as checking allergies, reviewing past medical history, or documenting the application of a splint, as well as for billing and insurance reimbursement purposes. The medical record grows and evolves from the patient's first contact with a prehospital medical provider to hospital discharge, rehabilitation, and beyond.

A medical record is a legal document. It is a log of all patient-provider interactions. This log is invaluable as a protection for the patient as well as the provider. Many people have access to the documents the provider generates, including—but not limited to—billing personnel, police, medical personnel, and insurance companies.

Benefits of Proper Documentation

Remember back in training when you read a case study? Somehow, no matter how obscure the authors tried to be, "rales" was always an easily identifiable symptom. By seeing the key words, "rales," "lung sounds wet bilaterally," "crackling," or "bubbling," you knew that congestive heart failure (CHF) was not far behind. These key words triggered an automatic response in your head that equated the written description with a diagnosis and a course of treatment.

Now, remember the first time you set foot on the ambulance? Remember your first CHF call? Not until your instructor suggested that the lungs were wet did you even understand the clinical presentation of CHF.

This is the first benefit of thorough, prompt documentation. By taking time to gather your thoughts and write your clinical impressions, you might see something that you may otherwise miss. Normal pulse, low blood pressure, and a calm demeanor may not mean much at first, but when you see these observations in the same paragraph as the mechanism of injury, such as a fall from 15 feet, you are more likely to recognize these as signs and symptoms of neurologic shock.

If the first benefit of accurately recording your observations and actions is that it assists you in providing care to the patient, the second benefit is that accurate documentation assists other health care providers who subsequently render care to the same patient. The main disadvantage that the trauma surgeon has in treating the patient is that he or she did not see the scene of the motor vehicle accident from which you pulled the patient. By completely describing the scene, using as many of your five senses as possible, you provide the necessary information to assist in the delivery of quality care.

In-hospital providers rely upon your initial fact gathering for aspects of care other than just diagnosis. The demographic information taken from the dispatch record may be the only indication of the comatose patient's residence, thus giving staff a place to start when attempting to contact the patient's family. Also, the impressions created from documentation regarding a patient's living conditions may be the only indication that social services are needed. For example, your documentation regarding an elderly patient may help identify if that patient is being neglected or abused by a caregiver at home.

Finally, from a risk management perspective, the most important benefit of adequate documentation is the protection that the record provides. The medical record is a legal document that is admissible in court under most circumstances. Most disputes do not appear in court until several months or years after the call, so you cannot rely on your memory alone to get you through a trial. By using the medical record, you can honestly and accurately discuss your actions in the courtroom.

Ideally, proper documentation will prevent a lawsuit from progressing past the initial filing. A medical record that is complete, thorough, and indicates care consistent with regional protocols and standards of care may bar a suit from proceeding past the investigative stages. Conversely, if your documentation is incomplete and fails to indicate care that was provided according to your protocols, you have reason for concern.

Consequences of Poor Documentation

One potential consequence of poor documentation is that an injured patient may claim that you breached your duty in providing care. Used effectively, the main piece of evidence that proves or destroys such a case is the medical record. Although the testimonies of witnesses and other health care providers are valuable, most juries place greater weight on the written medical record because it is less fallible and subjective than an individual's memory in personal testimony.

There are several reasons why so much emphasis is placed on medical documentation. First, it is presumed to be a true and adequate representation of the patient's care that was created contemporaneous to when the treatment was delivered. The impressions that were made, the results of diagnostic tests, the status of the patient, and the interactions that occurred during the care are all reported in the narrative of the patient care report. Due to the checks and balances of multiple authors contributing to a medical record at various stages of the patient's care, the authenticity of clinical representations made within a record is deemed to be high.

Second, the document is secure. Because so many people are involved in its creation, altering a document after the fact is difficult. Once the document has been created, hospitals, physician's offices, EMS agencies, and insurance and billing contractors have very specific procedures they must follow regarding how the documents are processed and stored. Your EMS agency's legal and administrative staff should be able to provide you with the specific procedures your agency has delineated for retaining EMS reports.

Finally, medical records are permanent. The document is created in some fashion that ensures its longevity. Most hospitals have secure backup systems for record storage, such as electronic or photographic copies.

Rules of Documentation

Because all providers who encounter a medical record can add to the document, there are some basic rules and assumptions that every health care provider must adhere to when documenting. You may wish to consolidate these rules into a systematic approach for documentation. Uniform use of the same documentation system will create consistency in evaluation and treatment of your patients, which will ultimately create additional reliability in your skills as an EMS provider.

Never assume that you are the only one who will see a record. Records are available to all providers involved in the care of a patient. Accordingly, your written report may be used and referred to multiple times during a patient's course of treatment. To prove this point, stand in an emergency department and watch a patient's chart. Within a few minutes, several people will have touched it—from the station secretary who adds the laboratory values that just came in, to the nurse who records a medication that was administered, to the physician who documents a physical examination, to the admission secretary who documents the patient's insurance information, to the technician who stops by to jot down the latest vitals. The record is a constant source of activity.

Never assume that you can:

1. Ignore negative findings on the chart.
2. Hide information on the chart.
3. Change information on the chart.
4. Delete information from the chart.
5. Falsely add information to the chart.

Always promptly document everything. This is a two-part rule. The first part deals with the time in which you wait to actually document information. The longer you wait, the more you forget. The more you forget, the greater the liability exposure you incur.

The second part of this rule, and probably the most important rule of EMS documentation, is the idea that "if it was not documented, it was not done." Years after you've completed a call, the only way to accurately and credibly recount the treatment you provided, such as whether cervical-spinal precautions were taken, medication allergies were assessed, or oxygen was administered, is to have such actions clearly documented. It is extremely difficult to convince any jury that you performed a particular action if you haven't documented the action.

One of the most common mistakes made in prehospital care documentation is the assumption that if something was not seen or not done, it does not need to be recorded. Legally, this is a false and dangerous assumption. Documentation of pertinent negative findings is just as important as documentation of positive findings. Hindsight is always better than foresight. Documentation of pertinent negative findings may, for example, help prove that a medication that was later considered necessary for treatment was not indicated while you were treating the patient. If you do not document the pertinent negative findings or note why a specific course of action that may have been indicated was not followed, the legal assumption would be that you did not fully assess the patient to adequately rule out or confirm a particular type of treatment. For example, if you are an EMT-B called to a patient who reported that he wasn't "feeling well" and you transported that patient without calling for advanced life support, and it is later determined that the patient suffered a "silent myocardial infarction," it would be extremely helpful for you to have noted on your report that the "patient denied chest pain, shortness of breath, and stated no cardiac history."

If you suspect that a patient is being abused, you must report and document this suspicion. When documenting abuse, objective language should be used as opposed to subjective. For example use "patient presented with bilateral bruising on upper extremities" as opposed to "patient had marks consistent with being grabbed forcefully on both arms." Detailed descriptions should be documented without creating bias in the description. The documentation guidelines should be the same as for the documentation of any other injury in the patient's record. In addition to documenting the abuse, note to whom suspicion was reported. In many jurisdictions, EMS providers are mandated to report elder and child abuse. This means that failure of an EMS provider to report suspected abuse cases to the appropriate authorities could result in civil penalties, including fines and loss of certification.

Dealing With Electronic Documentation Systems

Many EMS systems are starting to use electronic records. These records may be in the form of a handheld computer or a truck-mounted laptop computer. These computers rely on special software that base their design on the traditional paper run reports. The information that you enter into the computer is then stored in a database. Depending on the system, you may be required to download the information into a central computer system or it may automatically transfer to a central processor.

There are many advantages to using this type of system. One advantage is that the information is entered in a uniform format by everyone in the system. The information can then be processed and used for multiple purposes. For example, your actions can be automatically compared with the protocol for the patient's chief complaint for quality assurance purposes. In addition, the equipment you used on the run can be subtracted from the inventory automatically, and new supplies can be automatically ordered. Many EMS systems are enjoying greater efficiency from automated systems.

However, automation does have its risks. The fear of public disclosure of confidential information through computer hackers has inspired federal legislation governing the use of electronic records. According to the Health Insurance Portability and Accountability Act (HIPAA), all medical records are subject to strict federal regulations and oversight. This federal regulation is designed to protect the intentional or unintentional disclosure of private medical information. Ask your EMS administrator if your electronic record system is consistent with HIPAA regulations.

Regarding your daily interactions with electronic recordkeeping, remember that electronic records are designed to maintain the same standards as paper records. Just as with paper documentation, you do not want to completely erase incorrect information. However, with electronic documentation, you may need to correct errors in a special way. For example, you may need to electronically draw a line through the wrong information or highlight the information that you want to change.

All electronic records should be treated in the same fashion as paper records. Do not leave computer screens displaying patient information so

Legal Practices

1. Always attempt to document during and immediately after a call. Delaying documentation creates room for errors.

2. When documenting, do not use abbreviations that are hard to read or confusing. Complicated abbreviations are one of the leading causes of medical errors.

3. Do not leave patient records out in an open place. Although some facilities may have an inbox in which EMS providers are to place PCRs when they drop off a patient, just leaving the report in an accessible place, out and open to the public, may be a breach of confidentiality. Ideally, hand the report to the nurse or physician to whom you transferred care instead of leaving it in a general EMS PCR bin.

that bystanders can see what you are typing. Do not leave computers unattended with open patient records. Make sure that you use a password feature and that the password is not simply a stock password to which everyone has access.

Conclusion

EMS providers should consider documentation as important as their hands-on medical skills. The patient's record is a legal document that paints a picture of the interactions you had with your patient. Using a standardized documentation system that incorporates negative as well as positive findings for all patients creates a concrete, objective record of your interactions with your patients. Doing so not only reduces your liability as a health care provider, but may also facilitate better outcomes in the continuum of care.

You Be the Judge

Discussion

It would be extremely difficult for you to prove to a jury that you successfully intubated the patient because there is no documentation to support your claim. You and your partner can both testify as to your recollection of the facts, and you can testify that you always routinely check for accuracy and patency status post intubation, but the only documented fact the jury would have is that the tube dislodged and the patient suffered. If you cannot produce the piece of tape that you wrote your facts on, no jury would give credence to that explanation of events. Producing prior and subsequent run sheets that illustrate your routine practice of checking for status post intubation accuracy and patency may even harm you. The plaintiff's attorney could use those run reports to argue that because you do document these actions when they are completed, lack of documentation of such actions on this call illustrates that the actions were not taken. The only hope you may have is if there are recorded ambulance-to-hospital medical control radio tapes that are consistent with your version of the facts. However, even if such tapes exist, the quality of the audio may not suffice or you might not have provided medical control with the exact words a jury would want to hear to be convinced of your credibility.

Chapter 12

Insurance

You just started your own ambulance company. A local hospital offers to pay for your first ambulance as a sign of support. While handing over the check, the president makes a joke about how having friends on the street is good for business. You think twice about this comment, especially after the president gives you a wink and a pat on the back. You decide that he is just joking. A month later, your company gets a letter that the hospital is being investigated for violating the Stark regulations. You review your records and notice that 90% of your transports were taken to the hospital that paid for your ambulance. What is your liability?

Health care is a highly regulated industry. The delivery of health care is influenced by the ability to control, predict, and afford various risks. Although regulations are developed in an effort to control these risks, the ultimate control of unwarranted risks is achieved through the use of insurance. Health care providers use insurance to protect themselves against liability and to help pay for services. Patients purchase insurance as a way to secure access to care without experiencing significant economic repercussions. The government uses insurance as a means to purchase health care services for citizens, as well as to regulate the delivery of health care. Health care providers need to recognize the role insurance plays in the delivery of health care in order to be aware of opportunities to gain economic incentives and avoid potential liability for the violation of regulations.

Insurance and Risk

Insurance is a process through which risk is calculated and controlled. By purchasing insurance, a person is making a calculated gamble that the amount in premiums that he or she will pay will be less than the cost of the expenditures that would be incurred if he or she did not purchase the insurance.

Insurance companies can only make a profit if they have enough customers. Using the law of averages, insurance companies know that with a sufficiently large customer base, the premiums collected, in addition to the interest made from premiums that were invested, will cover the expenses that the customer base will incur in health care costs while still providing them with a profit.

The insurance business relies on the law of probabilities and the concept of diversification to remain solvent. To illustrate these concepts, imagine that you have a rich uncle who says that he will bet you $100,000 on a coin flip. You have a 50% chance of winning this bet. You also have a 50% chance of losing. These are not great odds. However, if you spread out the bets by betting $100 on a coin flip 100 times, thus giving you the opportunity to win all 100 bets for a total of $100,000, you are much more likely to come out ahead (or at least even). A similar theory for increasing earnings applies to the insurance business: A large customer base diversifies any extraordinary costs over the entire customer base.

When a person or business is covered by an insurance policy, the insurance company is liable for covering any expenses that may arise under the terms of the contract on behalf of the insured. It is important to note that through a process known as subrogation, an insurance company may seek to recover the expenses they paid if there are extenuating circumstances. For example, if you are in a car accident, your insurance company may pay your claim immediately, even though another party is at fault. However, the insurance company may seek reimbursement for the claim paid to you from the liable party as a result of a subrogation claim.

Insurance as a Payer of Health Care

Health care insurance, whether it is private or government-based, constitutes a majority of the health care purchasing dollars within the United States. This form of payment is governed through contract law as well as the specific laws that directly govern insurance. When you purchase an insurance policy, you have entered into a contract with the insurance company. They must provide you with service, according to the terms of the contract, for as long as you pay the premiums. The terms of the contract, however, can be complicated and burdensome.

State governments have regulated the insurance industry for the past 60 years in an effort to avoid harmful situations, such as bankruptcy of an insurance company that would prohibit the company from paying out legitimate claims. Therefore, most business decisions that affect the provision of insurance services must be approved by the state. The state, in an effort to ensure solvency of the insurance industry, may permit various provisions that limit or constrict services to an individual consumer in order to protect the overall consumer population. For example, in many jurisdictions, if a consumer files a claim on his or her homeowner's insurance policy, providers are permitted to refuse to grant that person a new or renewed policy. A similar approach is taken with medical policies. Many complex medical procedures are not covered on medical policies, whereas less costly (and less effective) procedures are.

In addition to regulating insurance, the government also provides health care insurance. On the federal level, the government, through the Department of Health and Human Services, operates the Medicare program. This is an entitlement program that was started along with Social Security in response to President Roosevelt's New Deal program after the Great Depression.

The Medicare program consists of two parts. Part A provides coverage for hospital services that are rendered on an inpatient basis. Everyone older than age 65 is automatically enrolled in Part A, and they do not have to pay any fees as long as they or their spouse paid Medicare taxes while they were working. Part B provides coverage for outpatient services, including the care provided by a personal medical doctor. Participation in Part B is optional and requires the patient to pay monthly premiums. In order to be eligible for Part B coverage, one must be at least 65 years old. Premiums are usually taken out of monthly Social Security, Railroad Retirement, or Civil Service Retirement payments, or they are billed directly to the patient.

In contrast, the states (with the help of federal monies) operate the Medicaid program. Medicaid is designed to provide health care services to a state's poor and medically disabled citizens. The benefits and eligibility requirements differ among the states. Whereas Medicare is viewed as an entitlement program that senior citizens have earned from their years of service to the country, Medicaid is viewed as a right of poverty-stricken or medically disabled Americans to obtain adequate health care. Originating within welfare programs, Medicaid provides a different set of rights and benefits than Medicare provides.

Regulation of Insurance

Traditionally, the regulation of health care services was thought to be a state function, meaning that only states had jurisdiction over health care issues. However, because the federal government is a payer of health care services through Medicare and, to some extent, Medicaid, it can enact various legislative provisions and regulations that influence the delivery of health care services, as well as the laws and regulations of individual states. Although federal regulation may not dictate the educational requirements or credentials necessary to practice medicine, it may address the methods or resources used to provide the care, which would ultimately impact the provision of EMS.

For example, the Emergency Medical Treatment and Active Labor Act sets forth specific criteria that Medicare and Medicaid participant hospitals must apply to all of their patients, regardless of the patient's Medicare or Medicaid enrollment. These laws primarily govern the transfer of a patient from one facility to another. Failure to abide by these regulations may result in hefty financial penalties as well as civil liability.

Other significant federal regulations that influence EMS providers are the Stark regulations. The Stark regulations are federal laws that provide a framework within which health care businesses can operate. Under these laws, which are commonly known as the "anti-kickback provisions," any act that encourages or influences a patient to seek care from one facility rather than another—whether intentional or not—is prohibited. In an attempt to reduce costs and eliminate fraudulent Medicare claims resulting from the unnecessary transport of patients in ambulances to facilities offering such incentives, the government has created regulations that range from limiting the stocks that health care providers may purchase to restrictions on where, when, and how ambulances can restock supplies from receiving hospitals, and limiting whether emergency departments may provide food for EMS crews.

Enforcement of the anti-kickback laws has become a priority for the Department of Justice and the Department of Health and Human Services. A violation of these laws is considered fraud and abuse by the government. Under these federal provisions, not only can the cost of a fraudulent claim be recovered, but also penalties and jail time may be imposed, depending on the circumstances. The government recovers millions of dollars each year in fraud and abuse cases.

EMS providers are particularly at risk for liability in fraud and abuse claims. Although most of the liability rests on the managers, owners, or administrators of EMS systems, you cannot assume that you will not be subject to the penalties of fraud and abuse cases. The easiest way to avoid liability is to contact medical control or follow your local department's protocol for determining the facility to which you will transport your patients. Keep in mind that amenities that you may receive from a hospital, including free or discounted meals, free supplies, or a comfortable EMS crew room, may be viewed as an enticement that caused you to take a patient to a particular facility instead of the one you should have transported to per protocol.

Recently, a large metropolitan hospital settled a case with the government for a significant amount of money. The government claimed that the emergency department of the hospital provided food, including pizza, sandwiches, and soft drinks, for incoming EMS units. It was demonstrated that when food was provided, the number of patients brought to that hospital from EMS crews grew significantly. As a result, the hospital earned additional revenue from the increased census numbers. It was determined that the free food was an illegal enticement under the anti-kickback regulations.

Private insurance companies may also place policy-specific regulatory requirements on the practice of health care providers. For example, primary care providers may be required to only refer patients to certain specialists or prescribe certain medications. These regulations are a part of the terms of the coverage and reimbursement contracts that an insurance company has with the patient and the provider. This may affect your job as an EMS provider in that you may be required to fill out specific paperwork or obtain physician signatures on documentation in order for the ambulance transport to be reimbursed. Your EMS system should keep you updated on the required paperwork and information necessary for billing purposes. Failure to acquire the appropriate information, paperwork, or signatures may prohibit reimbursement to your EMS system. This may also cost patients out-of-pocket expenses that would have been covered by their insurance if pre-authorization procedures were followed. Such oversights regarding paperwork may even be legitimate grounds for disciplinary action against you, including dismissal from your agency.

Insurance as a Protection

Insurance not only plays an important role in paying health care providers for services rendered, but it also is important in protecting the providers. Malpractice insurance is used by health care providers to avoid the fiscal repercussions of liability for negligent acts.

Malpractice insurance operates in a much simpler fashion than health care insurance. The health care provider pays a premium based on the risk associated with the provider's practice area. High-risk practice areas such as obstetrics and brain surgery, in which the potential for harm to a patient is high, are covered by the insurance company at a higher required premium than lower-risk practice areas such as dermatology or geriatrics. Additional information, such as past allegations of negligence or past disciplinary actions, may also raise a provider's rates.

Within the field of EMS, malpractice insurance seems to be an under-used resource. There are various reasons why EMS providers do not appear to participate in malpractice insurance as much as other medical professionals. Considering that a significant number of jurisdictions provide some form of immunity for EMS providers, the benefits of malpractice insurance may not outweigh the cost of the premiums. Additionally, because most EMS providers are certified (as opposed to licensed) and work under the medical license of a physician, the physician's malpractice coverage may cover the EMS provider's actions.

Malpractice insurance for EMS providers may be more applicable in jurisdictions where EMS providers are licensed and work under their own authority or in states where immunity for negligent actions is barred or nonexistent. In most cases, malpractice insurance for EMS providers can be purchased at a relatively low cost. The benefit of having malpractice insurance can be great because defending yourself in a negligence lawsuit can result in substantial costs that far exceed your financial resources. Without

---

Legal Practices

When purchasing an insurance policy, pay close attention to whether the policy is based on *claims made* or *occurrence*. A claims made policy is a policy which must be in effect on the date of the filing of the claim. For example, a rescue call takes place on February 25, 2001. A claim is made against the insurance company on January 3, 2002. A claims made policy would dictate that your insurance premium must be paid through January 3, 2002, in order for the insurance company to exercise the policy's coverage.

An occurrence-based policy must be in effect on the date of the incident or the event giving rise to the claim. For example, you had a policy in effect for the calendar year of 2001. The event in question occurred on December 9, 2001. Although you may not have renewed the policy when the claim was made in July 24, 2002, your policy would still offer you protection. If possible, it is preferable to obtain an occurrence-based policy.

malpractice insurance or immunity, you are susceptible to losing all of your possessions, as well as possible bankruptcy, if you are named in a lawsuit.

There are additional benefits associated with malpractice insurance. Some insurance policies may provide legal representation for its policyholders in the case that their policyholder is named in a lawsuit. Some insurance companies may also provide lectures or in-services to assist you in maintaining a proficiency in regulatory or legal matters affecting your practice as an EMS provider.

After you have obtained provider coverage, the insurance company assumes responsibility for paying any claims made against you under the terms of the policy. As a covered provider, you should note that the malpractice coverage may not cover grossly negligent acts and usually does not cover intentional torts, civil rights violations, or criminal liability. If an insurance company investigates a claim and determines that a claim paid fell outside of its coverage scope, you may be sued by the insurance company in a subrogation claim to recover the monies paid on your behalf.

Conclusion

The delivery of health care involves risk. There is risk in regards to whether your department or agency will be adequately reimbursed for the services you provide, which ultimately creates a risk as to whether your department will be able to afford to compensate you. There also exists a risk that you may be found liable for negligent patient care. Insurance may serve as a form of protection for situations when, despite careful risk management, an adverse event occurs. However, keep in mind that although insurance protects, it can also restrict, regulate, or complicate the delivery of care. Understanding how the insurance industry works and affects your practice within the EMS system may assist you in managing your risk as a health care provider.

Legal Practices

1. When performing an interfacility transport, do not categorize a transport as needing a higher level of care than the patient truly needs. For example, do not label a trip as advanced life support (ALS) simply because you have a paramedic on board, unless the patient truly needs ALS intervention. This act is called up-coding and is illegal.

2. As of January 2002, the Federal Office of the Inspector General (OIG) published a new safe harbor provision for restocking ambulances with equipment provided by a hospital. In this "safe harbor," the OIG allows restocking if it is completed under an arrangement with the hospital in which supplies are paid for by the EMS agency at fair market value or supplies that were used to treat an emergency patient are restocked (even for free) at the time of delivery of such emergency patient. You should check to see whether the arrangements with your local hospitals fall under these safe harbor provisions.

3. When documenting a patient run, you should never falsely add services that you did not provide. Document the patient's condition and the equipment used honestly. Failure to do so can lead to severe penalties under a fraud and abuse claim.

You Be the Judge

Discussion

Your liability in the situation described at the beginning of this chapter depends on several factors. Are there other hospitals that offer comparable services in your service area? Did your crews ever bypass these hospitals to bring patients to the hospital that donated the ambulance to you? Did a patient ever request to be brought to another hospital but was brought to the hospital in question regardless of his or her request? Are you or your crews receiving any other benefits or services from this hospital, including items that may appear to be very minor, such as free meals, flu vaccinations, and supplies? Are transports to this hospital billed at the same rate as transports to other hospitals? Are all federal, state, and private insurance reimbursement laws, rules, and regulations being complied with in your billing processes? Are patients that you transport to this hospital given any type of incentive (financial or otherwise) to request transport to that facility? Does the president or any other executive of the hospital have any role or say in the management or operations of your ambulance company? Are any of your full-time employees also part-time employees of the hospital (or vice-versa)?

All of these and other issues would be examined by the OIG in order for the government to determine whether you have violated any of the Stark fraud and abuse regulations. If you are found to be in violation of these statutes, you may face civil fines or even criminal sanctions (such as imprisonment), you could lose your government certification as a Medicare and Medicaid provider, and you may be required to refund all monies remitted to you by federal, state, and private insurance carriers, facilities, or patients. Essentially, you would be forced to permanently close your business. Regardless of the findings, you would need to provide the OIG with sufficient documentation and other evidence to answer all of their questions. Preparing such documentation requires a huge time commitment and, undoubtedly, expensive legal counsel. Finally, even if you are cleared, your start-up ambulance company may not be able to recover from the negative reputation associated with being a target of a federal investigation.

Chapter 13

COBRA and EMTALA

You Be the Judge

You respond to a local construction site to care for injuries associated with a fall. Upon arrival, you find an unconscious worker. You begin to work up the patient when his supervisor comes to you and asks you to take the patient to a distant hospital that is covered by their insurance. You realize that the patient needs a trauma center. The closest trauma center is operated by a competing hospital. You tell the patient's supervisor that it is not up to you and that you need to take him to the closer trauma center per protocols. You call in for medical control to the trauma center. When they hear where you are calling from, they realize that the work site is a union work site. The hospital with the trauma center does not treat union people because the contract for the union's insurance is with the competing hospital center that the supervisor asked you to take the patient to in the first place. Medical control advises you to go to the union hospital, despite its lack of trauma facilities. Because medical control and the construction site supervisor suggested that you take the patient to the farther away hospital, you do. What is your liability?

The Consolidated Omnibus Budget Reconciliation Act (COBRA) and the Emergency Medical Treatment and Active Labor Act (EMTALA) provide and maintain open access to the health care system, regardless of an individual's economic ability to pay for emergent, necessary medical care. Adherence to these federal laws that enforce the general principles of access to care and nondiscriminatory treatment is not optional. Although the laws focus on hospitals, EMS professionals are not excluded from their far-reaching effects, particularly if they operate hospital-owned ambulances. This chapter serves as a resource for the inner workings of such legislation and addresses how EMTALA affects EMS.

A Need for Action

Nonprofit hospitals are required to provide charitable services as a condition of their tax-exempt status. However, in the late 1970s and early

1980s many nonprofit hospitals suffered severe financial losses because of the large amount of uncompensated care they provided. By treating uninsured patients with serious conditions such as cardiac problems, trauma, or obstetrical emergencies, many hospitals expended significant resources for which they were never able to get compensation or reimbursement.

After encountering such significant losses, some for-profit medical facilities found that if they turned the patient away at the door, or transferred the patient to a public, municipal hospital, they could avoid having to provide uncompensated care. This practice became known as "patient dumping." At the time, there was no clear statutory prohibition against such actions. This became a substantial problem for the uninsured population because care was not being rendered in a timely manner. Additionally, such patient dumping forced the already resource-deprived public municipal health care facilities to incur additional expenses that would not be reimbursed, ultimately forcing many public health care facilities to lose substantial amounts of money and, in some cases, to close. The closing of the public municipal hospitals created a health care crisis by denying underinsured and indigent patients access to care.

EMTALA Legislation

In an effort to stop patient dumping, **EMTALA,** (also known as the "anti-patient dumping statute") was enacted as section 1867 of the Social Security Act in 1986. Usually Social Security regulations address benefits that are applicable only to elderly populations, such as the federal Medicare program—health care benefits offered by the government. EMTALA, however, is not limited to Medicare patients. EMTALA specifically covers "any individual (whether or not eligible for benefits under [Social Security]) who comes to an emergency department." The law applies regardless of who has initial contact with the patient (a nurse, doctor, or clerk) and of whether such contact is with the patient or a representative of the patient. In addition, the law further dictates that EMTALA requirements are applicable to all areas and departments of the hospital, not just to the emergency department.

Although the substance of this legislation is medically related, the terms and definitions used in the text of EMTALA regulation are legal definitions. Therefore, the legal definitions of terms such as **emergency medical condition, transfer, stabilize,** and **participating hospital** that were established by the Health Care and Financing Administration (HCFA), the originators of EMTALA legislation, are extremely different from the definitions commonly used within the medical community. When examining EMTALA legislation, be aware of the precise legal meaning associated with these terms and how that meaning impacts the EMS field. If EMS providers do not understand the exact meaning of these terms, they may run the risk of unknowingly violating the EMTALA statute. It should also be noted that the federal agency that used to be known as HCFA has changed its name to The Center for Medicare and Medicaid Services, (commonly referred to as CMS).

Legally Speaking

EMTALA Federal law that guarantees medical coverage to any individual who seeks medical care from a hospital for an emergency medical condition.

emergency medical condition A medical condition manifesting itself by acute symptoms of sufficient severity (including severe pain) such that the absence of immediate medical attention could reasonably be expected to result in placing the health of the individual (or, with respect to a pregnant woman, the health of the woman or her unborn child) in serious jeopardy; serious impairment to bodily functions, or serious dysfunction of any bodily organ or part.

transfer The movement (including the discharge) of an individual outside of a hospital's facilities at the direction of any person employed by (or affiliated or associated–directly or indirectly–with) the hospital, but does not include such a movement of an individual who has been declared dead or leaves the facility without the permission of any such person.

stabilize With respect to an emergency medical condition, to provide such medical treatment of the condition as may be necessary to assure, within reasonable medical probability, that no material deterioration of the condition is likely to result or occur from or during the transfer of the individual from one facility to another.

participating hospital A hospital that has entered into a provider agreement with the government to provide Medicare or Medicaid services.

The primary targets for enforcing EMTALA regulations are the hospitals that participate in federal Medicare services. Almost every hospital in the United States participates in the Medicare program because the majority of health care expenditures are directly reimbursed by this program. Medicare income is one of the largest income sources for all hospitals. Additionally, a hospital's ability to participate in the state Medicaid program may be dependent on its participation in the Medicare program. By applying EMTALA regulations to all Medicare and Medicaid providers, the government covers most facilities where the underinsured or indigent populations may seek care. This, in turn, effectively addresses the patient dumping issue because a hospital's ability to participate in federal medical cost reimbursements depends on its adherence to strict policies that prohibit the transfer of or refusal to treat uninsured or underinsured patients.

When a hospital participates with Medicare and Medicaid, the law places full responsibility on the hospital for the compliance of its medical staff, on-call physicians, contracted emergency physicians, nurses, and other employees. The hospital is legally responsible for completing the medical screening examination of the emergent patient, as well as the appropriate transfer of such a patient. In addition, it is incumbent upon the hospital to determine and appropriately address the issues encompassing the means of a medically appropriate transfer to another facility. Although in most cases the hospital is ultimately responsible, the law still places responsibility on EMS providers to not knowingly participate in the transfer of patients if doing so would violate the EMTALA provisions.

EMTALA specifically deals with patients experiencing an emergency medical condition. But what is the legal definition of an emergency medical condition? According to EMTALA, an emergency medical condition is defined as "a medical condition manifesting itself by acute symptoms." However, the phrase "emergency medical condition" extends into the area of childbirth and labor, and places emphasis on, and greatly restricts, the meaning of "stability." For example, the EMTALA definition of stability for women having contractions says that all such women are legally unstable until they have delivered the baby and the placenta. Other provisions deal with nonobstetric-related medical emergencies.

Because the definition of an emergency condition extends to events that may occur anywhere within the hospital, EMTALA defines the emergency department in terms of function rather than in terms of an actual department of a hospital. The law refers to the function of emergency treatment as the determination of primary assessment and treatment of presenting patients within the capabilities of the hospital. The broad scope of this definition implies that the functions of an emergency department can be performed in many areas of the hospital and are not limited to the emergency department itself. Other areas in which emergency department care may be provided include the grounds of the hospital, the obstetric units, a hospital-based clinic, a hospital-owned clinic, the hospital's urgent care facilities, and the 24-hour assessment services of psychiatric facilities. Current regulations also extend these emergency department functions to ambulances that are owned and operated by hospitals. Accordingly, EMS providers must be familiar with such legislation and its potential impact on the workplace.

A large portion of EMTALA legislation focuses on the transfer of patients from hospital facilities. A transfer occurs anytime a patient leaves the facility alive and not against medical advice. Situations that are considered transfers under EMTALA regulations include treatment and release, discharge without treatment, referral to a private physician's office, referral to a preferred provider organization (PPO) physician or clinic or the patient's personal physician, and off-site testing at freestanding facilities.

How do EMS providers determine if the patient is stable enough for transport? Ultimately, it is the transferring physician's responsibility to accurately diagnose or secure as much patient stability as possible before allowing the patient to be transferred. At a minimum, a physical assessment by a physician—not the triage nurse—is required. Keep in mind that many patients require transfer in order to achieve definitive medical stabilization. Smaller hospitals in particular commonly lack resources that are desperately needed by the patient.

An appropriate transfer is one in which the transferring hospital provides medical treatment within its capacity that minimizes the risks to the individual's health and, in the case of a woman in labor, the health of the unborn child. Therefore, the transferring hospital must provide stabilizing care *within its capability* to protect the patient before *and* during transfer and must be fully cognizant of the skills and competence of the transferring ambulance service. A transfer may also take place if the patient is unstable and a physician determines that benefits of the transfer outweigh the risks.

Under EMTALA regulations concerning appropriate transfers, it is not a violation of the law if a patient is initially stable and this condition deteriorates en route. If the patient does begin to backslide, EMS providers have the education, experience, and equipment available to appropriately handle the situation. However, it is the responsibility of the transferring physician to arrange transport that takes the level of care available by the ambulance crew into consideration. The physician must use reasonable foresight to determine the appropriate level of care necessary for transport. EMTALA regulations are clear that the source of the deteriorating condition does not need to be cured at the time of the transfer but need only be stabilized before the transfer. The transferring physician is responsible for determining the patient's stability at the time of transfer; therefore, the physician is ultimately responsible for enforcing the statute.

Here is an example of how EMTALA regulations impact the transfer of a patient: A 52-year-old man comes to a rural hospital complaining of difficulty breathing. The patient has a history of severe congestive heart failure in addition to end-stage renal failure. The patient usually has dialysis three times per week, but a snowstorm forced him to miss dialysis this particular week. The patient is examined and it is determined that immediate dialysis is necessary; however, the rural hospital does not have the resources for this service. The emergency department physician arranges a transfer to a large tertiary hospital that can accommodate the patient's condition. To stabilize the patient before transport, the physician may intubate the patient and start some preliminary pharmacological interventions. This decreases the patient's likelihood of deteriorating into respiratory arrest. Despite this stabilization, the patient will not survive the transfer without the assistance of forced ventilations during the transport. In order to transfer the patient and comply with EMTALA regulations, an advanced life support ambulance is the most favorable form of transport because the patient is at risk for complications and may need someone to administer additional pharmacological agents. A basic life support (BLS) unit may suffice if no other unit is available because BLS providers can use a bag-valve respirator to continue the assisted ventilations as needed. A wheelchair van, however, would not comply with EMTALA regulations.

EMTALA regulations also apply to the receiving facility. The statute states that the receiving hospital must have the "available space and qualified personnel for the treatment of the individual." Further, the statute specifically states that the receiving hospital must have "agreed to accept transfer of the individual and to provide appropriate medical treatment."

EMS providers, at one point or another in their careers, become players in the execution of transfers. Many EMS providers work for agencies that deal exclusively with interhospital transfers of patients. When transferring a patient, make sure you receive all of the patient's medical records. Further, you have a duty to obtain a full report on the patient's condition. If a nurse hands you a sealed envelope of medical records and instructs you not to open the envelope, that nurse is violating the hospital's duty to properly transfer care and ensure appropriate care during the transport, which may violate EMTALA law. Without having access to the patient's medical records, which document past medical history, medications, allergies, and current condition and treatment, it may be impossible for you to assess the patient's level of stability upon transfer.

Regardless of EMTALA standards, as the medical provider for the transport, you also have a duty to ensure that the patient is stable for transport before loading the patient onto your stretcher. Should you arrive at the transferring facility and determine that the patient is too unstable for the transport, requires more advance medical equipment than your ambulance contains (for example, an IV pump), or requires the administration of medications that are not within your protocols, you must notify the transferring physician immediately. Under such circumstances, you may have the right to refuse to transport the patient. In addition, you have the option and responsibility to contact your agency's medical director and have him or her discuss the stability and transfer of the patient with the treating and transferring physician before you depart for the receiving hospital.

Occasionally, an EMS provider may be affected by EMTALA legislation in a second-hand manner when selecting "the closest, most appropriate" hospital for a patient. For example, it is 2 am. You are called to transport a college student with severe abdominal pains. The campus officials ask you to transport the patient to a hospital across town because that hospital has contracted with the college to handle all of the college's medical cases. Despite this request, you must transport the patient to the closest appropriate facility based on the patient's medical condition, not his or her insurance or financial status or other arrangements. If the patient is in acute distress, you should transport to the closest hospital equipped to handle such an emergency, even if that hospital is not part of the student's health plan. Transporting a patient based on financial rather than medical decisions is not only ethically incorrect, but it also may subject you to EMTALA-related legal ramifications.

Because of EMTALA, the receiving hospital must treat your patient and can only transfer the patient after he or she has been stabilized. If you are working within a hospital-based ambulance service and you

Case Study

Arrington v. Wong (1998)

On May 5, 1996, Harold Arrington was driving to work at approximately 11:30 pm when he experienced difficulty breathing. Upon arrival at work, one of his coworkers called an ambulance. When the ambulance arrived, the ambulance personnel noted that Mr. Arrington was "in severe respiratory distress, speaking one to two words at a time." The ambulance left the scene with Mr. Arrington at 12:24 am and headed to Queen's Medical Center, the closest medical facility. En route, the ambulance personnel communicated by radio to Queen's and discussed the patient's condition with Dr. Wong, one of the emergency department physicians. In response to Dr. Wong's question regarding which facility the patient is followed at, the EMS crew answered that the "patient is a Tripler [medical facility] patient, [but] being that he was in severe respiratory distress we thought we'd come to a closer facility." Dr. Wong responded that "if you start on the treatment with the basics and the nitro, I think it would be okay to go to Tripler." As directed by medical control, the ambulance then proceeded to the Tripler medical facility, five miles away from Queen's. The ambulance arrived at Tripler at 12:40 am. The patient coded at 12:42 am. Hospital personnel at Tripler attempted unsuccessfully to revive Mr. Arrington. He died at 1:17 am.

Plaintiffs filed a lawsuit in the United States District Court for the District of Hawaii on May 4, 1998 against Dr. Wong, his physician's group, the Queen's Medical Center, the City and County of Honolulu (operators of the ambulance service), and the individual EMS providers caring for Mr. Arrington in the ambulance. Plaintiffs filed their lawsuit in federal court under a cause of action based on the EMTALA law.

In this case, the court held that the radio communication between the emergency department physician and the ambulance personnel that advised the ambulance personnel to take the patient in severe respiratory distress to a more distant hospital did not provide a basis for prosecution under the EMTALA law because the patient did not "come to" the emergency department before being discharged or transferred.

bypass your hospital because you know that the patient does not have insurance, you can be held individually accountable for patient dumping. Further, be aware of medical control discovering the insurance status of the patient and then advising you to take the patient to another facility. This too can lead you to EMTALA litigation. If you feel it is in the best medical interest to bring your patient to one facility, and you believe medical control has diverted you to another facility based on the patient's insurance status, reiterate your request to go to the facility you feel is most appropriate and specifically state your medical reasons to medical control. If you are still directed to go to a different facility, document the incident, including your conversations with medical control, and turn the documentation into your department's administration. The administration will follow up on the case and determine if legal or other action is necessary.

Protecting Yourself

It is likely that you will be called in to testify in an EMTALA action, and that your own actions (or failure to act) may be examined. When a potential EMTALA violation is being investigated, the doors swing open to liability for all providers involved in the care of the patient. As you see from the

Case Study

Root v. New Liberty Hosp. Dist. (2000)
In this case, a patient sued a hospital in a civil cause of action alleging that the hospital violated EMTALA law when the hospital discharged the pregnant patient without properly performing the medical screening and stabilization required by the statute.

Although the hospital's emergency department was covered under sovereign immunity, the district court denied the hospital's motion to dismiss the complaint on that ground. The hospital argued that the EMTALA explicitly incorporated Missouri's sovereign immunity statute. The court held that although EMTALA adopted state standards for the determination of damages in civil enforcement actions, it did not incorporate state law that was unrelated to damages; therefore the state immunity statute did not apply. The court held that because the sovereign immunity statute was in direct conflict with the intent of EMTALA, the U.S. Constitution stated that the state sovereign immunity statute had to yield to the federal EMTALA requirements.

The hospital appealed the district court's decision and lost. Although state hospitals are exempt from EMTALA under current law, this case suggests that municipal or governmental health care providers, including EMS providers, are not immune from EMTALA actions, regardless of what a state immunity sections may provide.

Case Study

Hernandez v. Starr County Hosp. Dist.

In this case, a patient sustained a significant traumatic injury at work. Upon arrival, the EMS providers, who were employed by a hospital-based EMS system, found the patient unconscious. Before departing from the scene, the patient's boss directed EMS personnel to transport the patient to a different hospital than where the EMS providers intended to go. At no time did anyone request that the patient be transported to the hospital where the EMS providers were employed. The patient sued the hospital that operated the ambulance service under an EMTALA cause of action. The patient claimed in his lawsuit that his medical condition was adversely affected by the extra travel time it took to go to the hospital where the patient's supervisor told the EMS providers to take the patient. The court found that the patient "came to the emergency department" when he entered the ambulance.

However, because it was reasonable for technicians to follow the instructions of the person in charge at scene, they were not liable for the EMTALA violation of transferring before stabilization because they were following the request made by the patient (or a representative thereof). If the EMS providers chose the further hospital without a request from the patient's boss, they would have been liable.

decision in *Root vs. New Liberty Hosp. Dist.*, the immunity that you may be afforded in typical negligence cases is not applicable in EMTALA cases. Therefore, you must be careful not to violate EMTALA requirements.

Here are some suggestions on how to adhere to proper standards of care while avoiding liability under the anti-patient dumping statutes:

During an emergency transport:

1. Do not disclose socioeconomic or demographic information other than sex and age over the radio. Avoid terms such as "homeless," "street person," or "frequent-flyer."

2. Do not bypass a facility that can appropriately treat the patient's condition unless you are ordered to do so by medical control or are requested to do so by the patient or the patient's representative. In either circumstance, document the instructions given and the reason for your hospital choice.

During an interfacility transport:

1. Obtain a full report on the medical condition of the patient before transport. Ask questions of the staff of the transferring facility.

2. Ensure that you have the proper equipment necessary to care for the patient during the transport.

3. Ensure that your medical protocols and training encompass the scope of care required by the patient's condition. If the patient

requires a medication that you are not authorized to administer, you should not transport the patient unless you obtain express permission from your medical control or the transferring physician changes the order to a medication you have the authorization to administer.

4. Your paperwork for the transfer must include the informed consent of the patient or the patient's legal guardian.

5. Obtain certification of transfer from the transferring facility. Certification (a written document that includes the name and address of the transferring physician, receiving facility, and reason for transfer) is required by the statute.

6. Although simplistic, it is imperative that you are fully aware of where you are going and that your directions to the receiving hospital are clear. In an unofficially reported case outside of Detroit, Michigan, a private ambulance company agreed to transfer a patient from one hospital to another. While en route to the second hospital, the transporting ambulance got lost. During the transport the patient's status deteriorated and the patient died. Not only were the EMS personnel subject to a negligence lawsuit, but they also were part of an investigation under EMTALA.

Penalties for Violations

There are weighty penalties as well as personal liabilities attached to violations of EMTALA. Violations are subject to governmental investigation and actions such as fines or restriction of services. Penalties for hospitals and physicians include being barred from receiving Medicare and Medicaid benefits, as well as being charged up to $50,000 per violation. Typically, an EMTALA violation involves several infractions in a single episode, which means a hospital is exposed to cumulative penalties of several hundred thousand dollars if the government chooses to pursue the matter to the fullest extent of its authority.

EMTALA not only provides for governmental action, but can also give rise to civil actions. First, one of the most significant EMTALA sanctions is the creation of a private right of action for a patient (or a patient's legal representative) to sue hospitals for personal harm incurred as the result of an EMTALA violation. Second, a receiving hospital may have the right to sue a transferring hospital for all financial losses incurred by the receiving hospital as the result of an inappropriate transfer by the transferring hospital. By requiring certain hospitals to accept transferred patients, the law creates the possibility that hospitals requesting transfers could sue receiving hospitals that refuse to accept the patient. The receiving hospital could be determined liable for the direct financial loss incurred by the hospital requesting the transfer. Third, any violation of EMTALA based on discrimination also may result in referral to the Civil Rights Division of the Department of Health and Human Services (DHHS) and may be grounds for criminal prosecution under one or more of the federal civil rights acts.

Conclusion

In the past, EMS providers were caught in the middle of a financially-motivated hot potato game that consisted of unwanted, underinsured, or indigent populations being transferred from facility to facility without receiving the appropriate care. Such patient dumping was the catalyst for federal legislation that places stringent requirements on the interfacility transfer of patients. EMS providers are faced with situations that are governed by this complicated regulation on a daily basis. Improper actions may lead to significant liability for the provider and the provider's agency. Taking proactive measures that are based on an understanding of the law protects you and your agency from unwanted liability and may even enhance your standing as a valuable resource within your agency.

Legal Practices

1. Do not transport a patient from one facility to another without access to the patient's medical records. Regardless of whether you are transporting an emergency or nonemergency patient, you have a responsibility to review the patient's medical records. This ensures that you can appropriately treat the patient and that you can give an adequate report to the receiving facility.

2. Unless you are working in a critical care unit and you are taking a critical patient from one facility to another for the sole purpose of gaining access to life-saving resources that the first facility does not have, it is your responsibility to make sure that the patient is stable before transporting the patient from one facility to another. Transporting an unstable patient may be equivalent to assisting with patient dumping.

3. When giving a report to medical control or the receiving facility, do not disclose any socioeconomic or demographic information, outside of sex and age, over the radio. Avoid using terms such as homeless or frequent-flyer.

You Be the Judge

Discussion

The facts in the scenario presented at the beginning of this chapter sound very similar to the facts in the *Hernandez v. Starr County Hosp.* case discussed in the case studies. In that case, the court held that the EMS personnel were not liable for the EMTALA violation of transferring before stabilization because they were following the request made by the patient (or a representative thereof). If the EMS providers chose the farther hospital without a request from the patient's boss, they would have been liable. In another case discussed in this chapter, *Arrington v. Wong*, the court held that an emergency department physician's radio communication with ambulance personnel advising them to take a patient in severe respiratory distress to a more distant hospital was not actionable under the EMTALA law

(continued)

You Be the Judge

(continued)

because the patient did not "come to" the emergency department before being discharged or transferred, which is required by statute.

With these rulings in mind, you need to examine whether your situation can be included in the scope of EMTALA. Unless you are employed by a hospital-based ambulance service, you may or may not fall within EMTALA's jurisdiction. Assuming the government does find that you fall within the scope of EMTALA, the next question is whether the precedents set in cases such as *Hernandez v. Starr County Hosp.* and *Arrington v. Wong* would be enough to protect you from liability. Based on these two cases, it may appear that you would not be liable for an EMTALA violation, but this is not necessarily true. Although such precedent appears strongly related to the facts of your case, district courts are only guided by prior rulings in other federal districts, not bound by them. Even if your incident took place in the same district as previous cases that appear to support your case, a new federal judge may choose to disagree with his or her predecessor and come up with a different ruling. As long as the judge reconciled the facts of your case with the prior cases and his or her current interpretation of the law, such ruling would be legally acceptable and probably upheld by a higher court.

There is additionally one major detail that makes the facts in your case distinctly different from the two case studies in this chapter. In your case, a trauma center was bypassed in order to take a patient to a hospital that lacked trauma facilities. The legislative intent of EMTALA is to prevent patients from being deprived appropriate levels of service based on financial considerations. In this case, you are bypassing a trauma center to take your trauma patient to a hospital that does not offer trauma services based solely on the patient's insurance. This is exactly the type of action the EMTALA was enacted to prevent. It is most likely that a judge would rule that transporting to the hospital without a trauma center was indeed a violation of EMTALA.

Even if you, as a nonhospital-based EMS provider, are not named in the EMTALA action, you are likely to be called in as a witness in the government's case against the trauma center. There is also a high likelihood that regardless of the EMTALA action, you would be named in a negligence lawsuit for bypassing the trauma center. In your defense, you would have to testify to the fact that medical control directed you to the nontrauma center hospital. Because you believed your patient required the services of a trauma center, at bare minimum you should have professionally questioned medical control's decision by specifically noting that you felt the patient required trauma center services and thoroughly documenting the entire incident with special emphasis on your communications with medical control.

Bibliography

Arrington v. Wong, 19 F. Supp. 2d 1151 US Dist, HI (1998).

Hernandez v. Starr County Hosp. Dist., 30 F Supp 2d 970 (1999, SD Tex).

Root v. New Liberty Hosp. Dist., 209 F.3d 1068 (US. Ct. App. 8th Circ, 2000).

Chapter 14

Public Service and Interagency Relationships

You Be the Judge

You arrive at the home of a prestigious family to help a pediatric patient with shortness of breath. The father is a prominent businessman and philanthropist; the mother is a dedicated volunteer for numerous organizations. Upon assessing the child, who appears to be having an acute asthma attack, you notice a long, thin, bruise on the patient's back. Bruises are also present on the child's wrists and around the back of the neck. You feel that the bruises are evidence of child abuse. As you prepare to call child services, your partner comes in and stops you. Your partner tries to convince you that the parents are pillars of the community and that you should not interfere. In fact, your partner and the parents belong to the same house of worship. You decide not to report them. It later comes out that you suspected abuse on a call but failed to report it. What is your liability?

EMS is an ever-evolving profession that is dependent on others by nature. Throughout its short history, EMS providers have relied on hospitals, the police, and the fire service to work with them. Today, even though many EMS agencies stand essentially on their own, EMS providers are still dependent on a variety of other agencies, including a receiving medical facility, medical control, the Department of Health, police, fire, and social services, for the provision of medical care to the public. Although this setup may seem burdensome, a strategically designed network of shared resources facilitates effective public service. In addition, it allows the greatest flexibility in the use of various community assets. For example, one city or town may have a scuba team or a field communications truck that other cities or towns can use if needed. Many communities benefit from the use of the resources, but only one set of resources needs to be maintained. The mix of agencies involved in an EMS system requires great individual agency accountability, but allows the good of the public to be best served.

Public Servant or Medical Provider?

The EMS provider is one of the only members of the health care industry who wears two hats: that of a medical provider and that of a public servant. This can create complications as well as confusion in understanding the mission of the EMS provider, specifically when one of these roles outweighs the other. A good EMS provider, however, can blend these two roles smoothly.

You and other medical providers have certain shared responsibilities. You have obligations to your patients. You also have obligations to the industry. These include keeping your clinical knowledge and skills current and staying educated about the latest trends in the industry. You have a responsibility to facilitate development within the medical sciences through participation in clinical research. You also have a responsibility to become active in the regulation of medical practice through participation in advisory boards and disciplinary actions.

As a public servant, you serve an active role in the protection of lives. You have the authority as a public servant to engage in limited trespass, enter crime scenes to assist in medical care, use emergency devices, drive emergency vehicles, and educate the public about your abilities and services. You have a responsibility to act in a professional manner and, in doing so, foster and further enhance the trust that the public has given to you. You also have the obligation to report certain findings to other agencies.

Reporting Requirements

Because they are considered public servants, various state legislatures have designated their EMS providers as subject to certain reporting requirements. For example, an EMS provider is required to report a situation that may suggest the occurrence of a crime. This means that you may be required to notify state or federal agencies in the event you suspect a crime such as abuse.

In most—if not all—jurisdictions, suspected child abuse must be reported to the authorities. The pediatric patient is usually defenseless, and it is important to obtain an accurate mechanism of injury to coincide with the injuries that are presented. Child abuse is typically covered up by the abuser; however, because of unplanned, intimate caregiver-patient relationships that occur between children and EMS providers during emergency calls, parents may not have the time or ability to cover up the signs of the abuse. In this instance, parents may hover too closely or constantly answer questions on the child's behalf, effectively prohibiting the child from speaking. Signs of child abuse include multiple bruises or injuries in various patterns or locations, withdrawn actions, or hypersensitivity to physical examination.

Arising from the legislative intent of child abuse reporting requirements, abuse of geriatric and disabled individuals has also become a mandated reportable event in most jurisdictions. In many cases, geriatric and physically or mentally incapacitated patients are just as defenseless as children. As the eyes and ears of the emergency department, EMS providers are already aware that the information gleaned from the scene is extremely important. Just as a cracked windshield in a motor vehicle accident signifies potential head and cervical spinal injuries, inappropriate clothing, significant bruising, or physical unkemptness may signify abuse or neglect of a geriatric or disabled patient. Keep in mind that abuse of geriatric and disabled patients can occur within skilled nursing homes and mental health facilities as well as in private homes.

Depending on your local statutes and regulations, you may be required to report other types of abuse, such as domestic abuse. You may also be required to report other actions, such as gunshot wounds, narcotic overdoses, or sexual assaults. Some of these reporting requirements may be delegated to the emergency department. Check with your local laws and your agency's administration and counsel for the specific requirements that are applicable to you and your practice. Your agency should also be able to provide you with useful resources that outline the common signs of domestic violence, child abuse, and elder abuse. If you check your local phone book, most cities and states have domestic violence and abuse hotline services that can provide you with information on signs of abuse and the area's reporting mechanisms.

If you feel as if you may be required to report a situation, report all circumstances surrounding the call to the emergency physician and nurses on staff upon your arrival to the emergency department. Document on your run sheet that such a report was made to the accepting triage physician. You may even contact social services on your own, depending on the protocols in place within your department. States that have reporting mandates tend to have procedures in place that usually include preprinted forms to help facilitate the reporting of suspected abuse and neglect.

Although it is imperative that allegations of abuse or neglect not be made in unwarranted conditions, the well-being of the geriatric, disabled, or pediatric patient may solely rely on your documentation and notification to the proper authorities. When documenting medical information and the surrounding conditions of a call, use objective words rather than subjective descriptions. For example, state "patient's soiled clothing was found in piles on the floor, and there were several dirty dishes in the kitchen sink and on the table. No food was found in the refrigerator" as opposed to "patient's apartment was a mess and unfit for human habitation; patient obviously cannot care for himself." Objective details stand the weathering of cross-examination by defense attorneys far better than subjective adjectives, and allow for proper intervention to occur, if necessary. Additionally, although documentation found in official reports usually cannot be used as a basis for a libel or slander suit, using adjectives such as "horrible parents" greatly harms your credibility as an objective reporter of facts, and that may lead to your report not having the impact that it should with the courts or agencies that would attempt to correct the problems you discovered.

Most states that require mandated reporting have immunity statutes that completely protect an EMS provider from liability for any good faith reporting of a suspected abuse or neglect situation. Case law also states that a case brought against an EMS provider for liability and damages regarding a report of suspected abuse will not stand if it is found that no

Legal Practices
Your state law may require you to report abuse. It is essential that you become familiar with your department's standard operating procedures and state and federal laws regarding abuse.

abuse exists and the report was made in good faith. Keep in mind that the reporting to authorities must be made in good faith, and not out of malicious spite against an individual.

Working With Other Agencies

Various agencies assist EMS providers, including medical control, medical helicopter teams, the poison control hotline, and general social service organizations. Police departments often assist EMS providers in subduing unruly patients. They also provide protection by securing the scene from traffic; crowds; or hostile friends, family, or bystanders. Fire departments, if they are not a direct medical component of the local EMS response system, may assist in vehicle extrication and technical rescues.

EMS systems must be careful not to overuse scarce resources. Inappropriate use of a limited resource is detrimental to other patients who may really be in need of specialized care. This is particularly true with medical flight helicopters, critical care ground transport teams, tactical support and rehabilitation units, and limited advanced life support units. Improper use leads to insurance reimbursement problems. In addition, a lack of confidence in the EMS agency may develop within the community if advanced services are not available when truly needed. Constant use of a scarce resource indicates that policies and procedures must be reevaluated to determine whether the overuse is based on need or abuse.

Underuse of resources is another common concern in EMS. The personalities of EMS providers are such that they tend to function best when in total control of a scene. They may hesitate to call for help from outside resources. Rather than attempting to be the sole hero of a call, consider what other resources you may need. Discretion is knowing that you should set aside your ego and request assistance. Stand back from the scene and properly evaluate it. Do you need another ambulance? Do you need the Jaws of Life and a hazardous materials team? Are the medical conditions of patients so critical that one or more medical helicopters are needed?

It is also necessary to recognize your limitations on the scene and request assistance when it is needed. When you undertake an unnecessary risk, you endanger your life and the lives of your coworkers, and you decrease your ability to assist the people who require help at the scene. Thus, it is imperative that you keep in mind the adage of "establish a safe scene." You cannot be held liable for knowing that you do not have the proper resources to handle a situation and calling for additional help. This includes, for example, staging and waiting for clearance from the police before entering the scene of an act of violence, even if your patient is in critical condition.

A resource that has traditionally been underused by EMS departments is the Critical Incident Stress Management (CISM) team. The CISM team provides individual and group counseling to rescuers who have been exposed to traumatic situations such as the death of a young child or a fire that involved multiple casualties. EMS providers are human. They, like everyone else, are bothered by some of the horrible scenes they encounter. CISM teams provide counseling for posttraumatic stress disorder and grief. They are an excellent example of a resource that is available to help EMS providers when they need it.

Most departments provide CISM services to their members free of charge and on a completely confidential basis. Although EMS providers have a duty to themselves, their families, and their community to take advantage of this resource, the duty is often ignored because they assume that using such services stigmatizes them as weak or poor providers. This assumption can be physically and legally dangerous. If you are not physically and mentally prepared for each and every call, you may suffer physical harm. Further, failure to properly address job-related stress might hinder your ability to do your job properly. Such stress may result in sloppy work, which increases your potential for liability for providing negligent care.

Regardless of how frequently external resources are used, appropriate plans and procedures must be in place regarding their use. Protocols are virtually useless if they are not followed and reviewed on a regular basis to ensure that they are up-to-date and applicable. Protocols are readily subpoenaed and scrutinized within the courtroom, so EMS providers must be prepared to be held legally and ethically accountable for their on-scene behavior. Additionally, whenever a scarce resource is used for patient care purposes, medical control must be contacted.

Implementing protocols and procedures for extenuating circumstances on a scene enables a facility to function smoothly when such circumstances arise. For example, it may be established protocol to request police assistance for all psychiatric calls. If an EMS agency lacks the necessary protocols and procedures for extenuating circumstances, the agency may be found liable.

Protocols must be easy to read and understand, and they must be kept in an easily accessible location. Documentation should be maintained regarding all training activities. In addition to creating and distributing protocols internally, an EMS agency may wish to incorporate the agencies with which it works into the protocol development and dissemination process.

Mutual Aid

Mutual aid relationships occur when two or more EMS departments arrange to share resources within various communities should a particular EMS system not be able to handle a situation with its own resources. Communities routinely call on a neighboring city or town when they have a request for EMS, and all of their ambulances are already on calls. These agreements between neighboring departments and agencies to help each other out should be formalized, and specific protocols should be developed. Establishing such procedures not only assists with a provider's ability to provide adequate care to patients, but it also may help avoid liability for failing to involve necessary outside resources to provide adequate care.

Legal Practices

Using mutual aid to supplement your ability to provide care when you do not have adequate resources available is a necessary part of all EMS systems. Failure to include mutual aid and outside resource coordination policies and procedures in your agency protocols may lead to increased liability.

Mutual aid is a valuable tool in providing finite limited resources to multiple communities without extensive expense. Hazardous material training and response, for example, is a common shared resource in mutual aid agreements. Mutual aid agreements also include support for disaster situations. Many smaller communities share an advanced life support paramedic response unit while maintaining individual basic life support first responder or transport services.

Legally, you may have an obligation to create mutual aid relationships to supplement your ability to provide care. Failure to establish and maintain communications with potentially necessary resources limits your ability to defend yourself in a lawsuit that claims your EMS department was unprepared for an emergency.

A Resource Allocation Checklist

- Stability of patient: How stable is the patient? What advanced care is required? What immediate care is required?
- Necessity of care that exceeds available resources (eg, helicopter or trauma center): What are the medical benefits versus the risks of situations, such as waiting to transport your patient until a helicopter arrives or bypassing a local hospital to go to a regional trauma center?
- Anticipated time for transport versus status of patient: Will a delay in transport ultimately help your patient because he or she will obtain needed advanced care, or will it harm your patient by losing valuable time that could be used to get to the hospital? Should you start toward the hospital and attempt to intercept the advanced care unit, or wait on the scene until the advanced care unit arrives?
- Skill level of providers on scene: Are the providers on scene skilled and equipped to handle the incident, or do they require assistance? Are the providers basic life support EMTs or advanced life support paramedics?
- Availability of mutual aid or additional resources: Are paramedics or a helicopter from a neighboring city or town available? How long would it take them to reach your scene? From which direction are they coming? Could you start transporting the patient and attempt to intercept them?
- Medical control: Are there specific protocols in place for calling additional resources? Can you contact online medical control staff and seek their input regarding whether you should begin transport or wait for additional resources?

Establishing a Chain of Command

As we have seen throughout this book, liability is never solely placed on one party. All those involved in an incident may be liable, under one theory or another, for harm that occurs. Accordingly, whenever working with outside agencies, it is imperative to designate a chain of command before interagency relationships form on the scene of a call.

Within the protocols, address the chain of command. Recognize that one person or agency may not be appropriate for all command issues. For example, during a disaster, the fire chief may be appropriate to head operations;

however, a designated emergency physician, if available, would be the appropriate choice for medical care issues. The current public safety incident management trend is for police, fire, and EMS agencies to use an Incident Command System that uses an interagency Unified Chain of Command to coordinate response, operation, and mitigation activities. In order for an Incident Command System to be successful, all participating agencies must be involved in planning, training, and implementation. For more information on the Incident Command System contact your State Emergency Management Agency or the Federal Emergency Management Agency.

In creating agency or departmental protocols, check with your department's administration, legal staff, and medical quality assurance staff to ensure that all liability, patient care, and administrative and financial issues are appropriately addressed in your chain of command. Creating a chain of command that falls outside the scope of your liability coverage or falls outside permissible practice as regulated by state law may be adverse to your agency.

Finally, know your internal agency or department chain of command. This applies to all circumstances, from reporting requirements associated with abuse to operational procedures associated with disaster response. Just as you need to be familiar with your medical protocols in order to provide care within the terms of your legal duty, you need to know how to handle special circumstances.

Conclusion

You are in a special situation as an EMS provider. Not only are you a medical provider, but you are also a public servant. Juggling these two roles can be complicated and burdensome. However, you have a legal duty and responsibility to fulfill both roles. Although your duties require familiarity with your skills and resources, appropriate use of outside resources when necessary is also your duty. Knowing the resources that you have available and planning for the best use of those resources will ultimately assist you in providing the best care that you can to your patients and your community.

Legal Practices

1. Your state law has reporting requirements for various incidents. You should have a list of phone numbers and preprinted reporting forms with your equipment to facilitate your reporting obligations.

2. Be familiar with the CISM team that services your EMS organization. Try to speak with them on a regular, routine basis. Meeting with them on a proactive basis will make use of this resource easier and more effective after a critical incident.

3. Using mutual aid is necessary when managing an incident is beyond the scope of your available local resources. The following are factors that may indicate when mutual aid should be considered: (a) the stability of the patient, (b) the necessity of care that exceeds available resources (eg, helicopter or trauma center), (c) the anticipated time for transport versus status of patient, (d) the skill level of providers on scene, (e) the availability of mutual aid, and (f) medical control.

You Be the Judge

Discussion

Your liability for failure to report suspected child abuse depends on the laws of the state in which you practice. Chances are you would be liable. Most—if not all—states have mandated reporting statutes that require EMS personnel to report suspected child abuse to a specific agency such as Child Services, Social Services, or the police. Penalties for not reporting abuse range from civil fines to loss of certification or licensure. Failing to report suspected abuse is also considered a violation of most department and agency policies and would result in discipline up to and including termination. In addition to the statutory requirement for reporting, you may be civilly liable under a negligence action for not appropriately transferring care by failing to report your suspicion to the receiving hospital's emergency department physician or nurse assigned your patient's case. Finally, statutory and case law has established that an EMS provider cannot be held liable for any unfounded report of suspected abuse or neglect as long as the report is rendered in good faith.

Glossary

abandonment   Occurs if a medical provider has entered into a patient-provider relationship, and the medical provider either transfers care to a person of lesser training, does not transfer care to any other provider, or stops providing care for the patient.

affirmative defense   A defense that is raised in the answer that, despite the truth of the facts of the complaint, excuses the defendant from liability; common examples of affirmative defenses include assumption of risk, contributory negligence, and self-defense.

answer   The defendant's written response to the plaintiff's filed complaint.

arbitration   The presentation of a disagreement to an impartial person or panel (agreed to by both parties) in a forum other than court, with the understanding that the decision reached by such arbitrator or arbitration panel is final.

assault   Any willful attempt to threaten to inflict injury upon another individual, coupled with an apparent ability to do so.

battery   The unlawful touching of another individual without permission or excuse. Battery may occur despite good intentions if care is provided without the patient's consent.

burden of proof   The duty of a party to substantiate an allegation to avoid the dismissal of that issue, or to convince the trier of facts regarding the truth of a claim in order to prevail in a civil or criminal suit.

cause of action   The legal basis for a lawsuit.

certification   Evidence of level of training; the formal assertion of some fact.

civil action   A lawsuit brought by an individual (the plaintiff) against another individual, corporation, or entity (the defendant) seeking to redress (through monetary damages or other court orders) harm that the plaintiff suffered as a result of the defendant's actions.

comparative negligence   The allocation of responsibility for damages to both the plaintiff and defendant based on the relative negligence of the two; the reduction of damages to be recovered by the negligent plaintiff in proportion to his fault.

compensatory damages   The cost associated with the actual harm caused that correlates to returning the plaintiff to the same standard of living and quality of life that he or she experienced before the alleged harm.

competent   Mentally sound and free from undue burdens or external influences to make a decision; the mental capacity to make a decision.

complaint   The initial document of a lawsuit filed in a court that describes the plaintiff's claims against the defendant.

contributory negligence   The actions of the plaintiff (the injured person) that fall below the standard to which he should conform for his own protection that may have led, in all or in part, to the harm allegedly caused by the defendant.

criminal action   A claim brought by the federal or state government on behalf of the citizens alleging a violation of the law that may result in the defendant being punished by fines, incarceration, or possibly the death penalty.

damages   Economic value of the harm caused to another; the loss, injury, or deterioration caused by negligence, design, or accident of one person to another in respect to the alleged victim's person or property; a monetary valuation of the loss sustained by the injured party.

defamation   The spoken or written falsehood by a defendant about a plaintiff that causes damage to the plaintiff's reputation or standing within the community; the publication of anything that injures the good name or reputation of another or brings him or her into disrepute.

defendant   The party against whom relief or recovery is sought; the party must defend or deny a cause of action.

dependent provider   A medical provider who provides certain care that falls under the same scope of practice as a physician, but requires medical oversight from a physician to render such care.

deposition   A discovery tool wherein factual and expert witnesses answer questions under oath in the presence of the respective attorneys; the testimony is recorded by audio, video, or a stenographer.

directed verdict   A request by the defendant to dismiss the case in favor of the defense on the basis that the plaintiff's attorney failed to meet all of the requirements for a valid cause of action.

discovery   A phase of the civil action in which each side has an opportunity to gather relevant information associated with the case from the opposing side.

dismissal with prejudice   A dismissal of a claim that is final and prevents the matter from being redressed in the future.

dismissal without prejudice   A dismissal of a claim on the grounds that it can be refiled within one year.

dissent   An opinion that disagrees with the majority opinion and is not a rule of law.

Do Not Resuscitate (DNR) order   A legally binding order for health care providers to not provide life-saving measures during a cardiac or respiratory arrest; created at the request of the patient or the patient's legal designee.

duty   A legally sanctioned obligation to perform a course of action originating from statutes, regulations, protocols, standards, policies, or case laws; if breached, the individual is liable.

emancipated minor   A person younger than age 18 who is legally recognized by the court as having the authority to make his or her own decisions; to be treated legally as an adult.

emergency medical condition   A medical condition manifesting itself by acute symptoms of sufficient severity (including severe pain) such that the absence of immediate medical attention could reasonably be expected to result in placing the health of the individual (or, with respect to a pregnant woman, the health of the woman or her unborn child) in serious jeopardy; serious impairment to bodily functions, or serious dysfunction of any bodily organ or part.

EMTALA (Emergency Medical Treatment and Active Labor Act)   Federal law that guarantees medical coverage to any individual who seeks medical care from a hospital for an emergency medical condition.

executive branch   The branch of the government that reports directly to the chief executive; responsible for executing, administering, and seeking court or administrative enforcement of laws and regulations; federal agencies overseen by the executive branch, including the FDA, DEA, and OSHA; state agencies include Departments of Public Health and EMS licensing and regulatory boards.

false imprisonment   The nonconsensual, intentional confinement of a person.

federal action   An action or responsibility of the federal government.

gross negligence   An act of negligence caused by actions that are willful, wanton, or a reckless disregard of a required duty or standard that result in an injury to the plaintiff.

health care durable power of attorney   A legal document originated and signed by the patient that names a specific person to act on the patient's behalf to make medical decisions, including the withdrawal or withholding of care, should the patient be incapacitated and unable to make the required decisions.

holding   The rule of law that comes from a case decision (also referred to as held or hold).

immunity   Protection from the consequences of litigation; the exemption from being held liable for damages; protection from being sued and having to pay damages; a right of exemption from a duty or penalty.

implied consent   The legal presumption that permission to render care in the patient's best interests is granted even though the patient is not competent to make an informed decision; occurs when a reasonable person in the same circumstances would be presumed to give consent.

incarceration   The loss of certain personal rights, including freedom through commitment to a penal institution, as a result of being found guilty, by a court of competent jurisdiction, of committing a criminal offense.

independent provider   A health care provider who may provide medical care autonomously under the authority of his or her own license, as opposed to operating under the control of a licensed physician.

intentional tort   An action, declared to be civilly wrong by the law, that is committed by an individual who knowingly intends to commit such an act.

interrogatories   Written questions from one party to another that must be answered in the discovery process.

judicial branch   The branch of government containing the courts that enforce the law and resolve disputes based on analysis of what the law means and how it applies to a given situation.

legislative branch   The branch of the government containing the legislature; the elected officials who write and enact laws.

libel   The publication of defamatory matter by printed or written words, by its embodiment in physical form, or by any other form of communication that has a potentially harmful characteristic.

licensure   The right to practice; the permission by competent authority to perform an act, which, without such permission, would be illegal, a trespass, a tort, or otherwise not allowable.

living will   A legal document originated and signed by the patient that provides specific instructions regarding the patient's wishes for the use of life-saving measures, including the withdrawal or withholding of care should the patient become incapacitated and unable to make or verbalize such decisions.

mediation   A process other than a trial in which the defendant and plaintiff actively participate in attempting to reach an agreement to a dispute; the proceedings are mediated by a neutral party.

medical practice act   The state legislation that grants legal authority to a health care provider to practice in that state and dictates the provider's scope of practice and practice environment.

medical record   A document containing confidential personal information regarding the health status of a person; created by a health care provider during the provision of medical care.

negligence   Failure to exercise the degree of care to which a person of ordinary prudence (a reasonable person) would exercise under the same circumstances that results in injury or damage to another.

negligence per se   An act or omission that is recognized as negligent as a matter of law because it is contrary to the requirements of the law or because it is so opposed to the dictates of common prudence that one could say, without hesitation or doubt, that no careful person would have committed the act or omission.

notice of intent   A letter notifying the defendant of the future possibility of the filing of a lawsuit by the plaintiff, which in some states extends the statute of limitations for a specified length of time; some states also require such notice if filing a suit against a state agency.

off-line medical control   Medical guidance, direction, or authorization provided by a physician before patient care is rendered; can be relied on in cases where online medical control is not available.

online medical control   Patient-specific medical guidance, direction, or authorization that occurs through direct, immediate contact between the physician and the EMS provider.

participating hospital   A hospital that has entered into a provider agreement with the government to provide Medicare or Medicaid services.

plaintiff   The party who files a civil action for recovery of damages, claiming he or she has been harmed by the defendant.

pleading   Written documents filed in court that set forth the plaintiff's cause of action and the defendant's grounds of defense.

police powers   The authority provided to states by the U.S. Constitution to adopt laws and conduct various acts to ensure public health and safety.

preponderance of the evidence   A degree of evidence that suggests that a person is more likely to be liable for harm than not; proof which leads the trier of fact to find that the existence of the fact in issue is more probable than not.

protocols   Written instructions that dictate necessary actions to be taken under various specific circumstances, usually developed by regional medical control personnel and considered to be the standing medical orders for that region.

punitive damages   Compensation assessed in excess of actual damages as a form of punishment for willful and malicious civil conduct.

scope of practice   The level and type of care that a provider may legally render based on state statute and local protocols.

settlement   A private agreement between the parties that resolves the lawsuit without judicial intervention.

slander   The publication of defamatory matter by spoken words, transitory gestures, or any form of communication other than those stated in the definition of libel.

sovereign immunity   Doctrine that limits liability of state and local government entities; based on the old English common law theory that one cannot sue the king (ie, government).

stabilize   With respect to an emergency medical condition, to provide such medical treatment of the condition as may be necessary to assure, within reasonable medical probability, that no material deterioration of the condition is likely to result or occur from or during the transfer of the individual from one facility to another.

standard of care   The degree of care that a reasonably prudent provider of similar certification level should render under similar circumstances.

state action   An action or responsibility of the state government.

statute of limitations   A period set by law that specifically limits the amount of time in which a lawsuit can be filed.

summary judgment   Pretrial or preverdict judgment rendered by the court in response to a motion by the plaintiff or defendant, who claims that the absence of factual dispute on one or more issues eliminates the need to proceed with the trial or to send those issues to the jury.

tort   A private or civil wrong or injury resulting from a breach of a legal duty that exists by virtue of society's expectations regarding interpersonal conduct rather than by contract or other private relationship.

tortfeasor   A person who commits a tort.

transfer   The movement (including the discharge) of an individual outside of a hospital's facilities at the direction of any person employed by (or affiliated or associated—directly or indirectly—with) the hospital, but does not include such a movement of an individual who has been declared dead or leaves the facility without the permission of any such person.

trial   A formal proceeding governed by judicial oversight that resolves a conflict between two parties.

voir dire   The process by which a jury is selected.

Index

Index